IT'S YOUR POWER PORTAL

IT'S YOUR POWER PORTAL

Take control of your vaginal health with herbal and holistic care

Kathie Bishop,
BA (Hons), BSc (Hons), MNIMH

INTO THE *wylde*

AEON

First published in 2022 by
Aeon Books

British Library Cataloguing in Publication Data

A C.I.P. for this book is available from the British Library

ISBN-13: 978-1-91350-488-5

Illustrations by Amaia Dadachanji, Jessica Jones & Claire Hartley

Typeset by Medlar Publishing Solutions Pvt Ltd, India

www.aeonbooks.co.uk

To all the men. May you raise fearless daughters who know their own bodies and aren't afraid to speak up about them.

And to the wild...

WITH THANKS

To my folks, Jane and Mike, for not dampening down their daughter, but feeding her instead.

To my beloved Mark, my ardent supporter, my love, who just gets it all…

To The Dreaming of Kate Bush, which accompanied me whilst I wrote.

Jo Farren, doula, herbal colleague and friend who shared her extensive knowledge around birth.

Amaia Dadachanji, herbalist and sistar of the wild, with whom I share many happy ramblings and who has contributed some gorgeous botanical drawings.

Claire Hartley, independent brand designer who brought Into the Wylde to life, and gave life to our female anatomy drawings too.

To everyone, attributed and anonymous, who has kindly donated their experience and experiences towards this book.

Lynayn Mielke for talking to me about five element acupuncture in relation to vaginal health.

Heidi Cresswell, for her encouragement and dedication to helping me get the title just right!

Rhiannon Levey, for all her unwavering support and wing-girl antics.

Susi Kaiser, my herbalist for many years, who lit a lamp.

Moira Bradfield, naturopath, teacher and founder of Intimate Ecology, for her incredible knowledge and her generous teaching.

Dr Emma Rees, for writing a cultural history of the vagina.

Sleater Kinney, Bikini Kill and all the other bands that gave me a kick in the pants when I was young.

To my patients and clients. You teach me, every day.

CONTENTS

INTRODUCTION   *xvii*

PART ONE: FANIMESTO: A MANIFESTO
Why is it important to look after your power portal?   2
How to use this book   3
Kathie's top tips for keeping your vagina wyldly happy   6
How to speak to your health care provider about
    your vaginal health   6
How to connect with your power/parts   7
The rules   7
A word about social norms   8
A word about FGM (female genital mutilation)   9

PART TWO: THE PHYSIOLOGY, MICRO- AND
MYCOBIOME OF THE VAGINA, THE VULVA AND
ALL THE ASSOCIATED PARTS
A word about 'balance'   14
The vulva   16
The mons   16
The labia   16

The clitoris   16
The vestibule   17
The urethral opening   18
The urethral sponge   18
The perineum   18
A word about vulval skin   18
It's not Hart's Line, it's mine: female anatomy named by men   19
The vagina   19
The hymen   19
More about the mucosa and discharge   20
Smell   21
Innervation   21
The vaginal microbiome   23
Cyclical changes to the vaginal microbiome   24
The vaginal mycobiome   25
The vaginal virobiome   26
How do your hormones fit in?   26
What is inflammation?   27
The neo-vagina   27

PART THREE: AGES, STAGES AND POTENTIAL ISSUES
WITH THE TISSUES
The female neonate   30
    How hormones affect the newly born girl   30
Childhood and pre-puberty   30
    What's normal?   30
    Signs and symptoms that may worry a parent   31
    Nappy rash   31
    Presence of foreign bodies   32
    Other dermatological issues   32
    Poor hygiene   33
    Pinworms   33
    Viruses   33
    Candida   34
    Bacterial   35
    Lichen sclerosis   35
    Other signs   35
    Some general advice for good intimate health for your
        female child   36

A word on consent   36
Adolescence and pre-menarch   37
The biologically fertile years   39
    A word on periods   39
    pH and testing   41
    Swabs   42
Common conditions during the fertile years   43
    Bacterial vaginosis   43
    Thrush   46
    Don't   49
    Cytolytic vaginosis   51
    Aerobic vaginitis   52
    Mollicutes   54
    Lichen sclerosus   55
    Lichen planus   56
    Cystic glands   58
    Vulvodynia, vestibulodynia, clitoridynia and pain   58
    Vaginismus   61
    Vaginitis   62
    Irritant contact dermatitis   62
    Allergic contact dermatitis   63
    Vaginal prolapse   64
    Inside out   65
    Fertility, pregnancy, miscarriage, birth and post birth   65
    UTIs and the urinary tract microbiome   68
    Pelvic inflammatory disease (PID) and
        pelvic congestion syndrome (PCS)   69
    How to spot pelvic congestion   69
    STIs   70
    A word about antibiotics   75
    What to do when symptoms or results are unclear and
        things just feel a little off   76
    The neo-vagina and likely conditions   78
How intercourse impacts vaginal health   79
    The sexual response, arousal, and libido   79
    A place for aphrodisiacs   82
    Orgasm   82
    A note on cervical health, smears, HPV, dysplasia, pleasure
        and de-armouring   84

Considerations   86
   Sexual health status and testing   86
   Lubricants   86
   Condoms   90
   Toys   90
   Hygiene matters   90
   Peeing after sex   91
   Smoking   91
   Obesity   92
   Immune health   92
   Menstrual protection   92
  Some considerations on hormonal birth control   93
  The emotional component to vaginal health   94
  Trauma   94
  The neo-vagina and penetrative sex   95
Peri-menopause into menopause   96
Menopause into post-menopausal   97
  Vaginal changes and what to expect   98
  Changes in the microbiome   99
  Freedom and power   100
  Talking to partners about vaginal health   101

PART FOUR: THERAPEUTICS

Limitations   106
Questions to ask yourself   107
Dosage forms   107
Tea and decoctions   108
Tincture   109
Sitz bath and washes   110
Compresses   110
Steams   111
Pessaries   112
The vagina is not a pocket   112
Other topical preparations—cream, ointments and gels   113
Abdominal massage   114
What do I mean when I talk about energetics?   114
Sex   115
Materia Medica   116
  How to use this section and how to choose your remedies   116

Hierarchy of therapeutics   117
How long to stay on the herbs and when to retake   118
What to do when everything reacts?   118
Getting to know herbs   118
Anti-inflammatory   119
    Chamomile   119
    Aloe vera   120
    Witch hazel   121
    Green tea   122
    Marigold   123
    Sodium bicarbonate (aka bicarbonate of soda)   124
Immunity   124
    Marigold   124
    Medicinal mushrooms   124
    Echinacea   125
    Vitamin C   126
    Vitamin D   127
    Prebiotics   129
    Probiotic   129
    Zinc   130
    Maca   131
Digestion and elimination   132
    Dandelion   132
    Cinnamon   133
    Chamomile   134
    Prebiotics—inulin   134
    Other ways to improve gut motility 134
    A note on senna   135
Mucous membrane integrity   135
    Broadleaf plantain   135
    Marshmallow root   137
    Bayberry   137
    EFAs   138
    Sea buckthorn oil   140
Nervines and aphrodisiacs   140
    Oats   140
    Chamomile   141
    Rose   141
    Ashwagandha   142

Vitamin B   143
Thiamin—B_1 144
Riboflavin—B_2 144
Niacin—B_3 144
Pantothenic acid—B_5 145
Pyridoxine—B_6 145
Biotin—B_7 145
Folic acid—B_9 146
Cobalamin—B_{12} 146
Damiana   147
Siberian ginseng   148
Mimosa   149
Jasmine and saffron   150
Hormonal   151
Fennel   151
Red clover   152
Phyto-oestrogenic foods   153
pH modulation   153
pH test strips   153
Probiotics as pessaries   154
Apple cider vinegar (ACV)   154
Sodium bicarbonate (aka bicarbonate of soda)   155
Antimicrobial   155
Barberry   155
Old man's beard   156
Garlic   157
Thyme   158
Vitamin C   159
Lactic acid gel   159
Probiotics as pessaries   160
N-acetyl-cystine   160
Sodium bicarbonate (aka bicarbonate of soda)   161
Anti-fungal   161
Aloe vera   161
Marigold   161
Garlic   161
Thyme   161
P'au d'arco   161
Olive   162

Oregano   163
Caprylic acid   163
Urinary   164
Olive leaf   164
Bearberry   164
Cornsilk   165
Buchu   166
Nettle   166
Cranberry   167
D-mannose   168
A note on UTIs   168
Other lifestyle considerations   169
Hygiene, clothing and toilet paper   169
Some considerations for pubic hair   170
Periodwear   170
Rowing and cycling   171
Low histamine diet   172
Dietary impacts on digestive health   172
Dietary impacts on immune health   172
Vaginal dilators   173
Blood glucose levels and how to go sugar-free or low-sugar,
   if you want to   173
Journaling prompts   177
Singing?   178
Other creative expression   178
Pelvic/women's health physio   179
Guided mediation to help your connection with your vagina   180
There are other therapeutics practitioners can use
(not mentioned in this book)   181
This woman's work   182

PART FIVE: MATERIALS
Glossary   184
Resources (all correct at time of going to print)   187
Condoms   187
Dental dams   187
Sexual health screening   187
Glass, ceramic and body-safe crystal dildos   188
Other pleasure tools   188

Intimate lubricants   188
Vibrating dilators for vaginismus   188
Professional practitioner bodies (for finding
    registered practitioners in different disciplines)   188
    Medical herbalists   188
    Naturopaths   188
    Nutritional therapists   189
    Somatic and sexual therapists   189
    Psychological therapies   189
    Abdominal massage therapies   189
    Pelvic health physiotherapists   189
Further help for people with cervical screenings   189
Great herb stockists in the UK   189
Supplements and products for self-guided purchase   190
Menstrual wear selection (many other brands exist)   190
    Period pants   190
    Sustainable organic disposables   190
    Discs and cups   190
    CBD infused   191
    Reusable cloth pads (including bamboo)   191
Charities working to prevent FGM   191
Recommended reading   191
And finally ... just a selection of the great and
    relevant therapists I know   192
References   193

INDEX   201

INTRODUCTION

Are you sitting comfortably? Then I'll begin. Or maybe it's best to start these things with a little discomfort, for that's so often how an interest in vaginal health starts.

So, let's try on that mantle of discomfort for size, see how it feels: Repeat after me: Vagina. Vagina, Vagina, Vagiiiinaaaaa.

Let it roll around your mouth, say it out loud, repeating in succession. Accentuate the vowels. How does it feel in your mouth? How does it sit in your bones? I'd love to say: 'see, it wasn't too bad was it?' But the reality is that there will be a large number of folk for whom that might feel, well, a bit self-conscious. A bit awkward. A hint of disgust? And that's ok. I want you to lean into your discomfort here. Breathe and relax. B r e a t h e. You're in safe hands.

Did you know that the accepted etymology of the word vagina comes from the old Greek word for sheath, or more specifically a sheath for a sword? And that gladius, meaning sword, was a common term for the penis. Slightly more acceptable is clitoris from the Greek word *kleitoris*, meaning door-tender, but it makes you realise just how far back the subjugation of female parts goes back. And it's so weaponised ... What do you make of that?

My name is Kathie. I'm a medical herbalist specialising in vaginal health, and, well, these are the kind of things I'm likely to come out with if you hang around with me socially. I was recently at a birthday party in a local pub. There were quite a few people I didn't know there, friends of my friend and her husband, as well as one of my oldest friends. A good mix of men and women. We were sitting outside and many of the women had gathered around a large table. We were asking each other what we did, learning about each other and where we could connect. Many were full-time mothers, others professional women, one was a psychologist. The drink was flowing and the late summer evening felt good. Then it got to my turn. It can go either way when we get down to it. I started talking about my work, both as a clinical herbalist and as the founder of Into the Wylde, a female, herbal-based intimate pleasure brand. The women were fascinated, crowded in a little closer, glowing just a little bit more together, got really curious, eyes sparkling. We started an interesting conversation around the politics of sex, the physiology of the vagina, and female body positivity. Everyone brought their own stories to the mix, their own viewpoints and were fascinated to learn a few facts that they hadn't previously known. The sharing of stories was great. It's not something we do very often, talking about our intimate health. Especially in beer gardens. But the more conversations we have, the more we normalise our bodies and the topic, releasing the fear and the shame.

And then the men, the husbands, the friends and the partners came over, and asked 'What are you talking about?'. Vaginas, we said. 'Urgh' was the response. My heart sank. 'Why "urgh"'?, I said, 'Don't you enjoy having sex? Weren't you there at the birth of your children?' But we'd lost them. They were turned off by the naming of our parts, and appeared not to be interested in the treasures to learn therein. Parts that hold an interesting place in our cultural imaginations. Parts that are at once desired but also derided. Parts that are simultaneously the ultimate taboo and the holy grail. Nightmarish images of 'vagina dentata' juxtaposing the deep holy reverence for the 'jade temple': The vagina as commodity and convenience in mainstream porn vs the birth canal for our children.

There's a lot of confusing stuff going on in society for us to get our heads around when it comes to vaginas, and I guess a beer garden late on one August evening in 2019 isn't necessarily ready for us yet.

But it really brought home to me a good couple of things. Firstly, the vagina needs a healthy dose of PR. Secondly, if good quality information about the vagina, its health, what to expect at different ages and stages, how to safely help ourselves and when to seek help, was easily accessible we would all be more empowered to take action. We could own the choices we make for the health of our bodies more easily, with pride. And that's where the idea for this book was born.

From the age of about 11, just after my menarche, I started a long, uncomfortable and deeply embarrassing relationship with thrush. I remember the first time on the GPs couch at that age, trying to pretend to myself I wasn't there, while they took a swab and sent it away for analysis. To wipe myself out of that picture. That first swab, plus countless others up to the age of 33, would come back with a positive result for *Candida albicans*—the yeast most commonly responsible for the majority of vaginal thrush infections worldwide. Over the years, becoming more frustrated, disillusioned and incredulous at my own body, I went on a journey, learning everything I could about how to reduce the occurrence and rid myself of thrush, consulting many allopathic and natural health specialists in this area, finally accepting that thrush was just something that was 'in me', like an invading force (which of course is what it is). I came to the conclusion that in order to deal with it I would just have to ignore it. In doing so I disconnected from that part of my body. Not so good, right?

In my 20s, whilst working in the arts, I decided to train as a medical herbalist. This had nothing to do with my own health history and everything to do with my own interests and hope for my future career path and work. Herbs and creativity are the threads that runs through everything I do and am. Through my own experiences and clinical work, it became obvious that vaginal health was the area I was set to specialise in. It's my passion. I'm passionate about ensuring that our experiences of vaginal health aren't marginalised, that everyone has a voice and is welcome to the table, and it is my passion above all to help women who have suffered repeatedly with bouts of vaginal issues: to reconnect them back to their bodies and creative power, with love and confidence, knowing that they have the knowledge and power to anticipate and manage their flare-ups and live an embodied life that they are the mistress of.

Will you join me?

PART ONE

FANIMESTO: A MANIFESTO

Icouldn't really set out a book like this and not have a manifesto for it. The term 'Fanimesto' came about through word play and spoonerism years ago (I'm funny like that) and found a home in my work. So let's set out this Fanimesto:

- This work seeks to connect women to their bodies; to give a greater understanding and working knowledge of their vulvas, vaginas and their intimate health, and a greater acceptance of their bodies.
- This work intends to empower women in and around their intimate health, giving language, knowledge and tools they can use themselves in the service of their health and comfort.
- This work intends to inform people of other genders about vaginas and their health, so that they can support us as true allies.
- This work intends to encourage the discourse around vaginal health; to normalise and break down the taboos associated with it, so that we can seek care when we need it and not be fobbed off or be told it's all in our heads.
- This work sets to break apart the unholy trinity of the three S's: Silence, Shame and Stigma and break out of patriarchal dogma.
- This work will give you the power to know your power, find your healing path and connect with the creatrix inside you.

I believe the world needs more women's voices, leadership and creativity. My part in this is in helping women to take control of their vaginal health and find their voice.

Why is it important to look after your power portal?

If you're someone with a vagina and you're reading this, you will almost certainly have some sort of relationship with this most intimate of places over the course of your life so far. It may have bought you pleasure. It may have brought you pain. It may have been involved in some sort of exchange with another person or a whole range of other commodities (commodities have a wide range of meanings here). It may have birthed your offspring. While acknowledging this, I'd like to propose a new way of thinking about your vagina: As sacred space. As the place where the divine creative feminine resides.

In many traditional cultures whose lineage hasn't been broken, the vagina is seen as the gateway to the pelvic bowl, that area in your body cradled by your hip girdle that houses your reproductive organs, uterus, ovaries and fallopian tubes, as well as bladder if you are assigned female at birth, which is a place of creative energy for a woman. Creative sexuality, spirituality, embodied power over your own destiny, as well as artistry. This isn't just about sex (although that can be part of it). And all of that is what I mean when I say your vagina is your power portal. It's the portal to all that power residing within you.

We need more feminine and creative energy in the world; the energy of collaboration over the energy of competition. And having a good relationship with the health of our power portals clears a channel for us to be able to express our creative energy in the world. Good vaginal health frees us from the discomfort that has often been hidden in silence, shame and stigma, stealing from our energy, leaving us in depression, anger, anxiety, repression, disconnection, desperation and shame. No more. Let's turn it around—it's your power!

We know 'pussy' is a powerful word in terms of sex. We know that the word 'cunt' is the most offensive word in the English language. Is it possible to make those words respectable in our culture, taking our privates away from that binary narrative of male vs female and rather looking at it from an energetic viewpoint? Reclaiming those words for our power portals.

As an interesting aside, did you know that in five element acupuncture there is an acupuncture point very close to the vagina, on the perineum, called CV1, that is associated with our ability to receive, as well as vaginal conditions, which are regarded often a subconscious expression of trauma, repression and shame? I think this is an interesting and possibly astute outlook: Are we comfortable to receive in life or do we repress those our desires and feel shame at the full personal expression of who we are? I don't think we should see this as negative, and if you don't feel this speaks some truth to you, that's ok too. After all, if we listen well enough, our body is talking to us all the time. And listening really is the key.

How to use this book

This book is one part call to arms, one part the hard facts that you need to know, and one part self-empowerment! I became a herbalist in part due to Led Zeppelin and partly because I believe in the democratisation of health. (Through Led Zep I discovered Sandy Denny and the world of folk music, which led to an interest and love of folklore and the utility of nature). While I know that a little knowledge can be a dangerous thing, to be able to recognise when something isn't right and to be able to take action into your own hands is not only empowering but is ensuring your safety too.

I've written this book to speak to anyone who has a vagina. This is not a work of gender essentialism and I have included sections on matters affecting neo-vaginas relating to trans-women too. This is important work because for too long women's health has been marginalised, doubly so for that of trans-women. This shouldn't continue.

I have also been aware that I didn't want this to be just my voice, but rather a diversity of voices, a platform for sharing experience. And so there are panels of prose and creative writing by other women, patients, colleagues who have given their time to voicing their experiences for you. Because to walk in another's shoes and feel what they feel gives us something of that experience, knowing that really, we are all one. To hear another woman's voice about her experience may encourage you to speak up about yours when it is needed to. You're not alone.

* * *

This book is divided into five parts.

You're currently reading the first part—it's a bit of a call to arms combined with some basic advice for how to look after your vagina. These concepts help create and maintain good vaginal health but are not routinely talked about, taught or passed on. Yet. Yes, let's be part of changing that. And you can apply them without knowing too much about the science behind it. If you already have robust vaginal health and all you take from this book are these points of power, then this section alone can work well for you. Pass on the tips. Talk about them with your friends, your mother, your boss at work, and tell your daughters, sister and cousins! Hell, tell your menfolk too! Let's normalise the conversation.

The second part is a good anatomical and physiological low down of what cis-gendered female-bodied adults have got down below. To intimately know your own terrain is empowering. You learn how it works and it gives you the language to use in case you need to seek medical help. It might even startle you to learn just how amazing the human body is.

The third part is where I go into many of the conditions and situations the vagina can find itself in at different points in life. I've arranged it by life stage to make it easier to find what you are looking for. Under each condition I have offered information about approaches and aims for treating the condition and given you advice about when to consult a health care professional. This is for your safety. Natural medicine can do a lot in regular folks' hands, but sometimes you need to speak to a professional to get the right treatment nailed.

This section also contains a reasonable amount of medical terminology. I believe that if we know the correct names for things, we can speak about them with confidence to our medical providers, ask questions and understand what they tell us back in answer. It allows us to uncover more about our health and take control of this vital area. I've added a useful glossary in Part Five—of not only words I have used here, but other words you may come into contact with on your journey to top vaginal health. Refer to it often and make friends with these interesting terms.

The fourth part might well be your favourite part … The part with all the magic, the part with the herbs. Here I go into detail about a lot of the herbs and other natural remedies and approaches that you can try for yourself and how to use them. This section on therapeutics explains the ways you can use the remedies in relation to the approaches and aims of Part Three, and the Materia Medica section goes into detail about the herbs themselves. The terms 'therapeutics' and 'Materia Medica' are the words that herbalists themselves use, so I'm inducting you into part of that world. Language is important and it holds power. Welcome to the inner circle.

Part Five is made up of a glossary, resources and references, which round out the picture.

* * *

Just a note to say that we don't cover cancer in this book. Treating cancer is outside the scope of practice of medical herbalists (although we can support the person with a cancer diagnosis). If you are concerned you may have signs or symptoms of cancer, please don't delay—go straight to get it checked out by your GP. They can either allay your fears or refer you on for further investigation. If you have a cancer diagnosis and would like support with a natural or complementary health therapy, please consult with a qualified professional. They can work alongside your more conventional treatments.

Kathie's top tips for keeping your vagina wyldly happy

As you're about to find out, the vagina doesn't need too much maintenance. It really doesn't. Despite what marketing and cultural discourse may have led us to believe, it really, really doesn't need too much day-to-day. Nature is clever like that.

A top way to keep your vagina happy is to leave her alone.

Avoid tight, synthetic clothing.

Only wash the outside parts with hair (this, as you're about to find out, is called the mons) with anything resembling a soap or gel of some kind, and only wash the vulva with water. Your actual vagina (the part that goes up inside) doesn't need soap, water, douching or anything. It's kind of got it figured out already. That is unless you keep getting intimate irritation. Then it might need some extra kind of help. But make sure it's the right kind (this book should help!).

In general, good advice around diet for vaginal health would be to balance your blood sugar by checking your intake of refined sugars and alcohols, avoiding processed foods and staying well hydrated (your whole body will thank you). Using the advice in this book, you can learn what is likely to be going on for you, when conventional treatment is needed, and the remedies you can try yourself. The Therapeutics section gives clear guidelines about how to start building your homemade remedy, and advice on when you may need to seek professional help. As with many aspects of life, you have to weigh up the risk-to-benefit ratio for any therapeutics, both conventional or natural, and sometimes you may need to speak to a professional to help you do that. It may be reassuring to know that many natural therapeutics can work alongside conventional treatment and, in many cases, can support their success.

How to speak to your health care provider about your vaginal health

When speaking to your health care provider about your vaginal health, use the anatomical names you are about to learn, as this will help you give information that accurately identifies exactly what is going on for you. Also, share with them how it is affecting you. Ask questions, ask for testing, ask all the options for treatment and ask for second opinions or to see different practitioners if you don't feel you are getting anywhere. Your body and health are yours, and no one knows more about what's going on for you than you do. You are the expert on that and your health care provider is there to help you to get to the bottom of what is going on. Remember that power dynamic. It's that way round.

How to connect with your power/parts

By growing in confidence around advocating for your vaginal health, you are connecting with those parts of yourself that may have been causing you issues for a long time. This is amazing. I often see people suffering with vaginal health conditions zoning out of that part of their body, dissociating from 'down there' as a way of coping. Coping can often be a needed strategy, but doing so can cut you off from this part of yourself—your sexuality, your creativity. While the aim isn't to have your condition form part of your identity (although this can happen with people), understand any vaginal pain or discomfort is part of you and your experience. Be open to integrating what your body is trying to tell you, listen to those messages and seek help for them if needed. There is nothing inherently wrong or dirty about you, and no reason to feel guilty, as though it is your 'fault'. Life happens and engaging with our bodies can simply be a great way to optimise our lives.

Towards the end of Part Four is a lovely meditation for helping you connect with your vagina: your power: your portal. Give it a go, along with the journaling prompts and creative ideas you can find before it. See if it works for helping you to claim your agency.

The rules

When looking at vulvovaginal health a good rule of thumb is to look at the colour, smell, quantity and consistency of the vaginal discharge. My advice is, make friends with yours. Get to know what it's like in health, during the different weeks of your cycle (if pre-menopausal), and keep this in mind. Your discharge is a great way to tell you when something isn't right and what that might be. You'll see it referred to a lot in this book.

You're probably most aware of a vaginal health condition when you suffer from pain, discomfort, or itching. These are three generalised symptoms people experience when something is going on. Don't ignore it. It's not in your head, and your body *is* trying to tell you something. While having these symptoms doesn't necessarily signify that you have something serious, please don't ignore it. And remember that your discharge can often provide great clues as to what's going on.

It is important not to fear our vaginal health and the signs and symptoms that it uses to communicate with us. Pathologising different aspects of our health as females is commonplace in society (the medicalisation of birth and the menopause—two totally natural, rather than pathological functions, *par exemple*). Instead, we can use our knowledge to help inform our choices and the language we use about them.

A word about social norms

Before we dive in up to our necks, I wanted to include a word about 'social norms'. What I mean when I say that is what we consider normal and acceptable in our society. And when I say society, I mean the vast majority, the 'middle of the road' that contains neither end of a spectrum. As I touched on in the intro, it's not really acceptable yet to talk about vaginas in an everyday social setting. This is a shame. The vagina has become stigmatised, but in reality it should be no more shameful or strange to talk about than any other anatomical part, such as an eye, a toe or a scapula. It's unhelpful not to be able to talk about the vagina as the vagina—making the vagina and anything that might be ailing it, embarrassing. It prevents people from getting help when they need it.

Calling the vagina cutsie names, as we are often taught in childhood, infantilises our vaginas and contributes to confusion in puberty when sexual feelings naturally arise. As I have already touched on, some of the most offensive words, certainly in the English language, as well as in many others across the world, refer to the vagina. Why should it be thus? It's time to reclaim these words and a sense of perspective about the effect language has.

Finally, as I end this part, a word on what I mean by vagina. By classic medical textbook definition, the vagina is a muscular tube connecting the cervix (which is the neck and opening of the uterus) to the external genitalia, in female mammals. However, as we are about to see, it is so much more complex than that. It's a whole ecosystem, affected by hormones, environmental factors, even emotions. This ecosystem is necessarily intertwined with that of the vulva (external genitalia) and the cervix and because of this, all these areas are carefully covered in this book.

In general, the information in the book has been designed to refer to natal (assigned at birth) aka 'cis'- vaginas. However, as explained above, I have included information applicable for neo-vaginas (assigned via surgery). There is still much more information needed to round out the picture in these cases. If you or someone you know could help to do this, please get in touch with Aeon Books and we will make updates if a second edition is published. Learning never stops.

What is worth taking away is that everyone's vaginas are as individual as the person, and neo-vaginas are no exception to that.

A word about FGM (female genital mutilation)

I wanted to include a short section here about what FGM is, for disambiguation and awareness purposes. This practice is still widely carried out throughout the world due to a mix of sociocultural factors, although the World Health Organisation has called it a violation of the human rights of girls and women. It is estimated that more than 200 million girls and women alive today have undergone the process. The following is directly taken from the WHO's page about it.[1]

Female genital mutilation (FGM) involves the partial or total removal of external female genitalia or other injury to the female genital organs for non-medical reasons, and is classified into four major types:

- **Type 1:** this is the partial or total removal of the clitoral glans (the external and visible part of the clitoris, which is a sensitive part of the female genitals), and/or the prepuce/clitoral hood (the fold of skin surrounding the clitoral glans).
- **Type 2:** this is the partial or total removal of the clitoral glans and the labia minora (the inner folds of the vulva), with or without removal of the labia majora (the outer folds of skin of the vulva).
- **Type 3:** Also known as infibulation, this is the narrowing of the vaginal opening through the creation of a covering seal. The seal is formed by cutting and repositioning the labia minora, or labia majora, sometimes through stitching, with or without removal of the clitoral prepuce/clitoral hood and glans. (Type I FGM).
- **Type 4:** this includes all other harmful procedures to the female genitalia for non-medical purposes, e.g. pricking, piercing, incising, scraping and cauterising the genital area.

Deinfibulation refers to the practice of cutting open the sealed vaginal opening of a woman who has been infibulated, which is often necessary for improving health and wellbeing as well as to allow intercourse or to facilitate childbirth.

Immediate complications can include:

- severe pain
- excessive bleeding (haemorrhage)
- genital tissue swelling
- fever
- infections, e.g. tetanus
- urinary problems
- wound healing problems
- injury to surrounding genital tissue
- shock
- death

Long-term complications can include:

- urinary problems (painful urination, urinary tract infections);
- vaginal problems (discharge, itching, bacterial vaginosis and other infections);
- menstrual problems (painful menstruations, difficulty in passing menstrual blood, etc.);
- scar tissue and keloid;
- sexual problems (pain during intercourse, decreased satisfaction, etc.);
- increased risk of childbirth complications (difficult delivery, excessive bleeding, Caesarean section, need to resuscitate the baby, etc.) and newborn deaths;
- need for later surgeries: for example, the sealing or narrowing of the vaginal opening (Type 3) may lead to the practice of cutting open the sealed vagina later to allow for sexual intercourse and childbirth (deinfibulation). Sometimes genital tissue is stitched again several times, including after childbirth, hence the woman goes through repeated opening and closing procedures, further increasing both immediate and long-term risks;
- psychological problems (depression, anxiety, post-traumatic stress disorder, low self-esteem, etc.);

FGM is mostly carried out on girls between infancy and age 15.

This information is shared here so we can be fully informed about exactly what is meant when we hear the phase FGM. There are many charities in the UK and around the world working to prevent FGM. I have listed some in the Resources section. If you are affected by this practice, some of these charities and organisations would be a good place to start.

PART TWO

THE PHYSIOLOGY, MICRO- AND MYCOBIOME OF THE VAGINA, THE VULVA AND ALL THE ASSOCIATED PARTS[2]

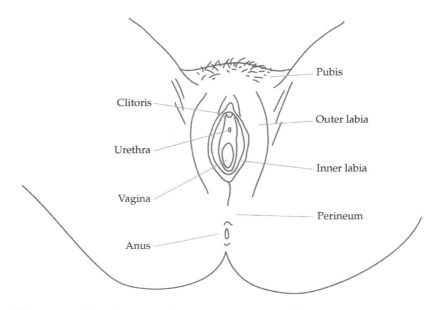

Pubis

Clitoris

Outer labia

Urethra

Inner labia

Vagina

Perineum

Anus

The external female genitalia

Now here's the bit where we name the parts and get a clear understanding of the space and terrain we are dealing with in this book. From this we will get clear reference terms that will be useful for the rest of our lives.

As you know I'm not a fan of cutsie nicknames that avoid the perceived embarrassment of naming parts, because it causes a lack of clarity which hamper our conversations with our healthcare providers, eventually leading to a true disconnection from our own bodies. I'm passionate about this because many of the women I encounter in my work are unclear about the true names of their intimate parts and what is actually 'down there', as though it is some mysterious terrain we have neither claimed for ourselves nor discovered. This adds to insecurities about whether something is 'right' about our bodies, and increases confusion about when something is actually wrong, out of 'balance' and needs our attention.

A word about 'balance'

It is both a great help and a great bugbear of mine to refer to the 'balance of the vagina', or rather the vagina being 'out of balance'. On the one hand, it is a great way to describe an overall impression of the state of health of the vagina in question. 'Balance' can refer to many aspects of vaginal health, such as the pH balance, the balance of the microbiome (bacterial colonies) and mycobiome (fungal colonies). However, it is also a great word to confuse and befuddle the general populous. Often when it appears on the internet, no one knows what it really means, no explanation is given, and it's often in a context that creates anxiety that something might be wrong with us and we need to buy a product to 'fix' us: We are 'out of balance' and therefore faulty. I am against that.

Back to physiology … As a child, teenager and younger adult, I was in the position of being too embarrassed to utter the word 'vagina'. However, and very relevantly, through my work and knowledge, repetition makes things normal. So let's name it and get to grips with what we've got.

In this book we will be talking for the main part about cis-female bodies who have passed through puberty, in that all the anatomical parts will be fully developed and present. We start from the exterior parts and move to the interior ones. In some sections we will also cover trans- or neo-vaginas.

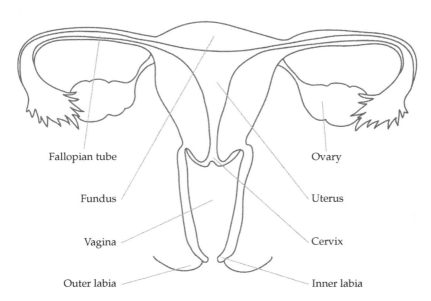

Fallopian tube

Fundus

Vagina

Outer labia

Ovary

Uterus

Cervix

Inner labia

The female reproductive system

The vulva[2]

As illustrated in this diagram, is often lumped in with the catch-all term 'vagina' because of laziness, embarrassment, ignorance and fear on society's part. It plays a large role in sexual pleasure (it houses the external part of the clitoris), but is also incredibly tough with its ability to heal and withstand childbirth.

The vulva is in fact the general term for the external female genitalia and is made up of:

The mons[2]

The fatty tissue and skin that is covered in hair, starting from around the pubic bone and down to where the clitoris hides inside. It forms part of the protective barrier protecting the entrance to the vagina.

The labia[2]

This is made up of the labia majora and the labia minora. The labia majora continues down from the mons to the vestibule area (the opening and surrounding area to the vagina) and has some fatty tissue and glands and can vary in size and length from person to person. The labia minora sit inside these. They do not have fatty tissue, but instead have erectile tissue, which can engorge with blood during sexual stimulation. The labia minora form part of the covering over the external clitoris, called the clitoral hood, which to some degree or other covers and protects the clitoris. The glans (the external part of the clitoris) is sited within the labia minora. The labia minora has many nerve endings that can greatly differentiate touch. They may or may not extend past the labia majora—it is entirely individual in each person and nothing is abnormal in this, nor a reason to worry.

The clitoris[2]

Much is being written about the clitoris now that more research (since the 1980s) has been carried out on this unique part of the anatomy. It is the only part of the body, male or female, that exists solely for pleasure, with over 8000 nerve endings sitting in a structure that is about 10 cm or more in length. Many of the nerve endings sit in the glans portion of the

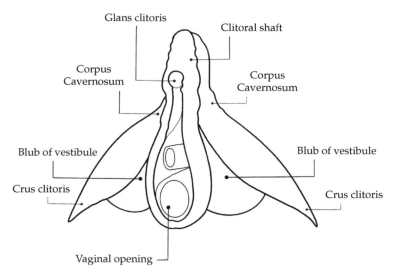

Glans clitoris

Clitoral shaft

Corpus
Cavernosum

Corpus
Cavernosum

Blub of vestibule

Blub of vestibule

Crus clitoris

Crus clitoris

Vaginal opening

The structure of the clitoris

clitoris, which is the externally visible section. The clitoris is the shape
of a 'Y' but with two sets of arms, 3–9 cm in length. The bottom point
of the 'Y' is folded over and forms the externally visible part, under-
neath the clitoral hood. It sits on top of the urethral opening (pee hole)
and the arms (two crura and two bulbs of vestibule) internally wrap
around either side of the vaginal opening and the lower section of the
vagina. The bottom of the 'Y' faces the front of the body, with the arms
of the top of the 'Y' facing the back of the body. All parts of the clitoris
are involved in sexual stimulation and are made of erectile tissue. With
this in mind, part of the clitoris is stimulated by penetrative sex and, in
fact, your G (Gräfenberg) spot is where this tissue comes closest to the
vaginal wall.

The vestibule[2]

The vestibule is the area inside the labia minora around the vaginal opening. It is external on the body, but the skin here is mucosal skin similar to that inside the vagina—it has no hair or sebum
secretion and the cells are filled with glycogen. In the vestibule there
are two sets of glands, one being the Bartholin's glands which sit

on either side of the vestibule at 4 and 8 o'clock (if you picture the vestibule as a clock face) and Skene's glands which actually secrete small amounts of prostate-specific antigen (also secreted in men from the prostate gland) and sit either side of the urethral opening. There is also erectile tissue in the vestibular bulbs, which sit on either side of the clitoris.

The urethral opening[2]

This sits within the vestibule area and is where your pee comes out. It is between your glans clitoris and your vaginal opening.

The urethral sponge[2]

Erectile tissue that surrounds and cushions the urethra. The posterior side sits closest to the vaginal canal and can be involved in orgasm, as we shall see later on.

The perineum[2]

This is the area of the skin between the vagina and the anus.

A word about vulval skin[2]

Vulval skin produces keratin, which helps to make the cells waterproof and to provide protection from damage and infection. The top layer of these cells is replaced approximately every 30 days. The mons and labial cells have sweat glands in them and have very fine and coarser pubic hair, which help to trap moisture and provide a barrier. They also have sebaceous glands associated with them that produce sebum, adding to skin conditioning and waterproofing, and sweat glands that become activated during puberty, releasing odour compounds that may have some role in sexual attraction.

All of the secretions combine to form a protective film known as the acid mantle. The pH of the vulva is 5.3–5.6, which is slightly acidic. The pH of the vagina is around 3.8–4.5, which is much more acidic (this is why you get bleached knickers). Where the skin of the vulva changes to that of the vaginal mucous, it is known as Hart's Line.

It's not Hart's Line, it's mine: female anatomy named by men

I don't know if you've noticed, but some of the names of the female anatomy are named eponymously after the doctor (normally male back in the days when they were still discovering anatomy) who officially 'discovered' it. It may have worked for them back in the day, but what do we feel now? Are we okay with that, or does it make us feel a little icky? Why not rename those parts anatomically rather than after men? Would that give us a greater sense of agency over our own bodies when talking to a medical professional?

The vagina[2]

As we've already covered, the vagina is the muscular tube connecting the vulva to the cervix. The muscular tube of the vagina is made up of smooth muscle, which is not under our conscious control, and may spasm (as may happen in period cramps or vaginismus). Lining the vaginal muscular tube are specialised skin cells called mucosa, which are secretary cells (other examples of mucous membranes are found lining the mouth, nose, eyelids, trachea, lungs, stomach, intestines, ureters, urethra and urinary bladder—mucosal cells aid lubrication!). The mucosa is arranged into folds called rugae, which may feel textured on contact with your fingers.

The combination of smooth muscle and the rugae-ed mucosa allows the vagina to be collapsed under everyday conditions, with the walls touching, but also to stretch to proportions big enough to deliver a baby.

The vagina is surrounded by a rich network of blood vessels, which deliver the nutrients for healing any trauma, such as vaginal delivery of a baby and to deliver the blood needed in sexual arousal.

The hymen[2]

Although it's not clearly defined as to why the hymen exists, it's probably a protective barrier, useful before puberty which produces protective mechanisms such as hair and acidic vaginal pH, to keep dirt out of the vagina where it could cause a very inflammatory response. It exists in the lower portion of the vagina and can be a partial covering, ring-shaped, have holes in it or be absent. It doesn't determine virginity.

More about the mucosa and discharge[2]

The mucosal layer is where the magic happens and is the main stage for much of what's to come in this book. It can be up to 40 layers thick, depending on hormone levels, and is constantly producing new cells— just about every four days! The cell turn-around is so quick because they need to protect against friction, provide adequate nourishment for the complex ecosystem of the micro- and mycobiome and to attach to bad bacteria and flush them out as they exit. They are hard-working cells that need continual replenishment. Mucosal cells are differentiated from the cells of the vulva by the fact they have much less keratin in them, making them less waterproof, and are filled with glycogen which is a sugar store that the *Lactobacilli* feed on. The fact that these cells are less waterproof than the cells of the vulva means that not only is the vaginal mucosa much more absorbent than other parts of the external body, but also that some fluid from the bloodstream leaks between the vaginal cells and forms part of the vaginal discharge.

The vaginal discharge (aka mucous) is a protective substance that acts as an important barrier between what is you and the outside environment. Components of discharge include: fluid pushed out from the blood between the intracellular gap junction between mucosa cells by blood pressure; secretions from the cervix, which change throughout the month according to hormone changes; secretions from the Bartholin's and Skene's glands; cells that have been shed from the vaginal walls; and products made by the vaginal microbiome. The discharge keeps the vaginal tissue moist and aids comfort (see the sections on menopause), and it is usual that most cis women produce anywhere between 1–4 ml of discharge a day. Clear, non-foul-smelling discharge is healthy and physiologically normal, even if produced in what may feel like copious amounts. If your discharge colour deviates from clear/milky to brown, pink, white, frothy, green/grey for a prolonged time please seek professional medical help.

Smell

While we are on the topic of what we may worry about as being normal, it's worth pointing out that vaginas and vulvas do have a smell. A healthy smell may be musky to some degree and can, anecdotally, be influenced by food you may have eaten. An unhealthy smell may be fishy, or yeasty, or one that can be smelt by others (in actuality, rather than you just being worried that it might be) when you are clothed and going about your daily life. If this occurs, you should certainly seek professional medical help. Every woman will smell slightly different, and this will be influenced by her individual microbiome, but rest assured it is normal and you shouldn't have zero smell or smell perfumed (please don't use scented products down there!). To have a smell is to be normal.

Innervation

The genital area is richly supplied by two nerve bundles, the pudendal nerve and the pelvic nerve. The pudendal nerve innervates (meaning to supply with nerves) the external genitalia, while the pelvic nerve innervates the deeper pelvic organs. These nerves transmit sensations as well as trigger any movement (such as the cervix moving higher in the vaginal canal during arousal, making way for potential penetration). There is always a plentiful nerve supply for any erectile tissue in the body.

When talking about the nerves of the female genitalia and reproductive organs, often the pelvic nerve is missed out. It innervates the deeper areas of the vagina, cervix and clitoris, the uterus, bladder and anus, the vestibular bulbs (erectile tissue, either side of the clitoris), the perineal sponge and the deeper part of the urethral sponge, as well as the deeper pelvic floor muscles. The pelvic nerve can respond well to the deeper thrusting/pounding of sexual intercourse, but only if there has been sufficient arousal to move the cervix up and out of the way, otherwise the cervix gets pounded and this can be a painful experience!

The pudendal nerve innervates the vulval skin, three parts of the clitoris, and the more superficial aspects of both the urethral sponge

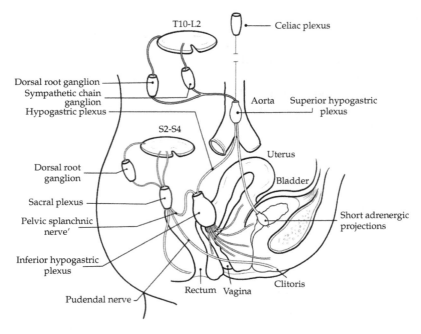

The pudendal nerve and pelvic nerve

and the pelvic floor muscles. These nerves respond to light, delicate sensations. Interestingly, the word pudendal comes from the Latin word *pudendum*, meaning 'to be ashamed of',[3] and has been used to describe the whole of the female genitalia. Does that feel familiar? This notion of shame goes back a long way and is deep-rooted in patriarchal cultures and language.

The two nerve bundles that enter the vaginal canal are called plexuses. The nerve plexuses then split into many smaller branches to continue to innervate the area. These nerves provide the experience of sexual pleasure and orgasm, the sensitisation and pain of some of the conditions mentioned further on, and the involuntary movement and signalling involved in arousal and childbirth. They are important to know about for these reasons and to know that surgery in this area, whether for medical, genital mutilation/cultural, or cosmetic reasons, can accidentally damage them—both because the nerve supply is so rich, but also through ignorance (the correct innervation of this area is often 'missed out' of anatomy textbooks[4]).

The vaginal microbiome

This is the part we are all starting to get very familiar with now in popular medical culture. Much has been written about the different microbiome sites of the body in the last few years, and the ones we are most familiar with are the gut and the skin microbiome. Interestingly, we rely on our microbiomes in a synergistic way for a variety of health benefits and there may be more synergistic bacteria cells in our microbiomes than we have human cells in our bodies!

Many take probiotics orally after, say antibiotics, thinking that they might beneficially affect their vaginal health. There is no evidence that probiotics taken orally translocate to the vagina through the gut, though there is evidence that they can via the faecal-vaginal route. I digress.

Now, we are familiar with the idea of the microbiome in general, but what about the vaginal microbiome? In health, the latest metagenomic (DNA) sequencing techniques have established that the vaginal microbiome can be made up of around 300 species of bacteria, viruses and yeasts,[5] and more are likely to be discovered over the coming years in this exciting and emerging research field known as vaginal microbiome mapping. In dysbiosis (disorder and ill-health), that number can increase and in fact, the higher the diversity of species the more likely it is that the microbiome is in a dysbiotic or infection state.

In health, the bacteria of the vaginal microbiome constitutes the first line of defence for us, by ensuring that invasive and harmful bacteria do not take hold and cause issues.[6] Some of the most helpful and well-known bacteria that make up a large percentage of the healthy vaginal microbiome are the gram-positive *Lactobacillus* species, known as *Lactobacilli*. This species of bacteria feed on the glycogen produced by the vaginal mucosal cells and produce lactic acid and hydrogen peroxide, keeping the vagina at its acidic pH of 3.8–4.5, which in turn keeps pathogens under control. This is good news. They also bind to the mucosa of the vaginal walls and help stop pathogenic species from inhabiting there.

There are four main types of *Lactobacilli* that we currently know about as being helpful in vaginal health: *Lactobacilli crispatus, L. gasseri, L. jensenii* and *L. iners*. Of these, *L. crispatus* is most implicated in eubiosis (healthy) vaginal states, and *L. iners* is known to become more prolific when a vaginal environment moves from being eubiotic to dysbiotic. This is a growing field of research and it is expected that more

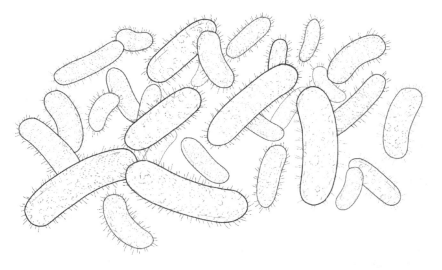

Lactobacilli

and more information will come to light over the coming years through the Vaginal Microbiome Project.

In 2011, Ravel et al.[7] studied the euboitic microbiomes of a group of almost 400 women, in equally weighted ethnic groups. This study determined that there are five community subtypes of healthy vaginal microbiome, each dominated by one of the four *Lactobacilli* (*L. crispatus*, *L. gasseri*, *L. jensenii* and *L. iners*) and one in which *Lactobacilli* were not dominant and yet still maintained eubiosis, albeit with a slightly elevated pH.

Cyclical changes to the vaginal microbiome

Menstrual blood is more alkaline than our vaginas, and so during our periods the normal environment in the vagina may be altered. The vaginal mucosal cells produce more glycogen after ovulation, due to peak levels of oestrogen, which may be used to feed opportunistic yeast cells to the point that they can cause a thrush outbreak. It's worth bearing in mind these two factors when thinking about your own patterns and note that the vaginal microbiome is a dynamic environment constantly in flux. In fact, hormones are one of the largest influencers on the vaginal microbiome!

It is also worth knowing that alongside the *Lactobacilli* many other types of bacteria reside there, such as Group B *Strep*, *E.coli*, *Psuedomonas*, which all need oxygen to survive, and others such as *Gardnerella vaginalis*, *Atopobium vaginaea* and *Prevotella* species which need to be in a non-oxygenated environment to survive. These and many others can normally live quite happily inside the vaginal environment as long as they are kept in check by the *Lactobacilli*, and it is normal for them to do so. It's when this gets out of balance (there's that word) that there may be an issue to deal with. More about this later.

Microbiome tests are now becoming more commercially commonplace and they can be bought online and used easily at home for DNA profiling. In fact, I use one such diagnostic service in my clinic when we are trying to work out what may be going on for a client in a complex or unclear picture. I believe these have a place in working out what might otherwise remain unfathomable when there are unresolved symptoms. However, there are two problems with this. Firstly, we have already established that the vaginal environment is a dynamic one and changes from day-to-day. If testing is done at the 'wrong' point, then a distinct picture of what is going on may not be made clear. Secondly, if used outside of a clinical setting, and not interpreted by an experienced clinician, wrong conclusions can be drawn, causing unnecessary worry and confusion to the person undergoing testing. As women, we are marketed many products aimed at quelling the fears we have been conditioned to have about our bodies through patriarchal messaging. Many of these products are superfluous at best, and, at worst, counterproductive to true vaginal health. We do not need yet another product to be added to the list of an already alarming number of concerns we've been told to have about our bodies, when not needed. There may be times when vaginal microbiome testing is useful. Always work with a clinician experienced in this area to work out when it is required and what the test can tell you.

A good rule of thumb is, only investigate and treat if you are experiencing issues. Everyone's microbiome is different and what is working for you, works for you.

The vaginal mycobiome

Integrated along with the vaginal microbiome is the vaginal mycobiome. Whereas 'micro' refers in greater part to the bacterial community, 'myco' refers to the yeast and fungal community. Until recently, research in this area was restricted to what could be cultured at the labs. However, with the emergence of tools such as genomics (DNA) sequencing, the complexity of the vaginal mycobiome is starting to be researched and discovered. Although vastly lower fungal numbers and species are encountered than microbial ones, they do make up an important part of the vaginal ecosystem. Due to previous research focused solely on *Candida* species, which are the fungal species mainly responsible for vaginal thrush, the rest of the vaginal mycobiome is poorly understood in comparison to the vaginal microbiome.[8] This area is likely to yield interesting information about the vaginal environment in the years to come.

The vaginal virobiome

Just as the mycobiome sits alongside the microbiome, the virobiome also inhabits the space too. This is where a variety of naturally occurring viruses sit, often happily in the vagina. In fact, some of the bacteria are under the control of the virobiome! Fancy that!

How do your hormones fit in?

Oestrogen is one of the key players in determining the nature of the vaginal tissues (plump or atrophic), the properties of the vaginal mucosa (glycogen levels) and the make-up of the microbiome. However, progesterone and testosterone (yes, women have testosterone levels just as men have some oestrogen too!) also play a role. They are involved in the female sexual response and libido, and testosterone and oestrogen are involved in helping to determine the health of the vestibule too.[9]

These three hormones also have an effect on pain perception as well. Research has shown that oestrogen levels have an association with 'feel-good' chemicals in the brain, and that that oestrogen and progesterone levels are inversely proportional to nerve conductivity of pain. As progesterone rises in the second half of the cycle, the threshold to pain drops, meaning that pain can be more easily felt. It has also been shown that testosterone confers a pain reduction benefit, possibly because it can reduce inflammation.[10] These things are worth bearing in mind when looking at the vulval and vaginal pain felt in some of the conditions further on.

What is inflammation?

Before we go any further, it's a good idea to have a reasonable definition in mind of what inflammation is so that you can recognise it without doubt when it occurs. The five cardinal signs of inflammation are redness, heat (feeling warm or hot to the touch), swelling, pain and loss of function. Inflammation is a response of the immune system, designed to bring healing components of the immune system to the site of tissue damage or injury. It can be a useful process for this reason, but if continuing for a prolonged time or if it becomes chronic, resolution is not found, and the symptoms cause great discomfort for the person involved.

The neo-vagina

For transgender people transitioning from male to female, and for females born with dysgenesis, which is an underdevelopment of the sexual organs (such as in Mayer–Rokitansky–Küster–Hauser syndrome or Rokintansky syndrome, both of which are congenital conditions), a neo-vagina can be created. For cis-females experiencing this, the options can be non-surgical self-dilation methods, or surgical interventions, including surgical dilation or vaginoplasty to create the neo-vagina using skin or intestinal transplants.[10]

In the case of people transitioning from male-bodied to female-bodied, the surgical creation of a neo-vagina, vulva and clitoris is often the last stage in a full transition and not every person transitioning decides to go to this stage.[10] For those that do, the successfully created structures are normally formed from penile, scrotal or intestinal tissue, and may require regular use of dilators for an extended period of time to maintain the depth and girth of the neo-vagina, especially if there is no regular penetrative intercourse occurring.

Like all areas on the human body, neo-vaginas will have their own microbial colonies and compositions living on the tissues there, but they will be different from that of natal vaginas (at birth female-assigned bodies), and they have their own set of considerations which will be covered further on.

It is also worth considering that a neo-vagina will have cosmetic concerns as well as functional concerns, which will be of interest to the person undergoing the creation of such. While the majority of this book refers to natal-vaginal health, I aim to cover some of the relevant topics for those with neo-vaginas, as I feel it is important to be of use to *all* those who identify as women.

PART THREE

AGES, STAGES AND POTENTIAL ISSUES WITH THE TISSUES

The female neonate[11]

In many books covering vaginal health, the female child is often never covered. That must be confusing for parents who may be seeking solid information on family health. Maybe it's because, as a culture, we don't like to focus on the sexual organs of children. I can understand why. However, sometimes 'needs must', as we look to protect and preserve the health of our children. Developmentally, as a foetus, the vagina starts as a solid tube, which then hollows out from the top (cervix) to the bottom (the opening) before birth.

In general, oestrogen levels are much lower in children than adults, and they are not affected by the same type of cyclical fluctuations that you get with a fertile-age woman, although they will fluctuate.

We currently don't know whether a female neonate is born with a sterile or colonised vaginal microbiome.

How hormones affect the newly born girl

After birth and for the first eight weeks of life the newly born girl is under the influence of maternal (the mother's) oestrogen that they experienced in utero, which initiates changes in the body, microbiome and the vaginal mucosa. It may mean that there is a presence of *Lactobacilli* in the vaginal microbiome, but this remains unproved.

This circulating oestrogen causes the labia major and minora to thicken, which closes off the vaginal opening to the external environment. No vaginal discharges are expected at this age, although in the first 14 days of life, due to the maternal oestrogen levels withdrawing, there can be a bloody discharge similar to a menstrual bleed. This can be understandably disconcerting for new parents. Oestrogen levels fall off after the neonatal period of eight weeks.

Childhood and pre-puberty[11]

What's normal?

After the initial eight-week neonatal period, oestrogen levels begin to fall. In fact, circulating oestrogen is lowest between the ages of about 3 and 8 or 9. This renders the vaginal mucosa of the newborn atrophic (reduced in size) in the same way a decrease of oestrogen does in a menopausal state. Biologically, this makes sense as the vagina is not needed for any reproductive or sexual function at this point. The labia major and minora become thinner than at the neonatal stage.

During this period, there can be some slight fluctuations in hormone levels, as may be implied by mood swings. However, overall this time in a female's life is considered to be one of low oestrogen levels.

Another effect of low oestrogen in childhood is that it renders the vaginal pH around 6–7. This is considered a more pH neutral environment, and is much more alkaline than adult vaginal pH. Also, due to low oestrogen levels, vaginal glycogen levels are low, meaning that there is much less proliferation of *Lactobacilli* in the childhood vagina. This creates a different microbiome profile with higher diversity of happy and not so happy microbes than you find in a healthy adult vagina, and lower immune defence than you get in adulthood. Bearing this in mind, it becomes understandable why issues may arise.

Signs and symptoms that may worry a parent

It's not uncommon for female children between the ages of 3 and 10 to get some vulvovaginal symptoms that may worry a parent. In most cases, the vulva is affected, but vaginal symptoms such as discharge may also be relevant.

Things to look out for include a red or scaly rash, swelling with possibly heat, a white rash, blisters, erosions or ulcers, plaques or patches of different looking skin and of course discharge of any sort. The difference between signs and symptoms is that symptoms can be felt and sometimes seen, whereas signs are clinical indications that can be tested for.

Nappy rash

Nappy rash appears as sore, red skin around the bottom and vulval areas (in a girl) that can extend to the tummy and thighs. It may also look swollen and be warm to the touch with red spots or bumps. It is this spread of symptoms and a lack of unusual vaginal discharge that may be useful in differentiating it from other things that might be going on. It's caused by prolonged exposure to a damp nappy, combined with friction from movement and ammonia products in the urine. Wearing anything containing plastic over this area may increase the problem as it stops air circulating. If the problem persists, it may become infected, which would be indicated by a rash that doesn't go away, with red or white pimples that may also be in the folds of the skin.

Infection may be bacterial, such a *Staphylococcus* or *Streptococcal* infection, but more commonly it is caused by yeast from the *Candida* species. We'll be hearing a lot about this yeast in this book. It's good to get familiar with it! It should be noted that aside from nappy rash would it be unusual to see *Candida* in a child. If it is present, further investigation into why is necessary!

Suggested treatments: To clear it, change nappies regularly, thoroughly clean and dry the area, allowing as much non-nappy time as is practical, expose the area to sunlight, and use barrier creams. If it persists, it can be assumed that an infection has taken hold, and you could try a gentle calendula cream from a 'herbal-friendly' pharmacy. If that doesn't shift it, it's worth going to see a qualified professional natural health practitioner for more targeted advice.

Presence of foreign bodies

Although the vagina is quite closed off in childhood, research has shown that 17.6%[12] of female children with vaginal discharge have a foreign body lodged in the vagina, such as crayons, beads, and balls of tissue paper. Children love experimenting and it's quite often that children will put small objects into small places. The nose is another, more common site. The discharge is often a brown colour with an unpleasant smell, due to the formation of bacteria, and is quite characteristic of this issue.

Suggested treatments: Removal is the best cause of action and antibiotics may be required.

Other dermatological issues

Other dermatological issues may include eczema, folliculitis, contact dermatitis, which can all present as red, irritated skin and/or a scaly rash. Aside from nappy rash, these can be caused by soaps, bubble baths, sand (if playing in a sand pit or on the beach), perfumes in wipes, certain materials and dyes in clothing. The best way to determine what might be causing it is removing all the factors listed above and, if needed, to reintroduce them one at a time so you can see what is the causal factor.

Suggested treatments: Bathing with anti-inflammatory herbs (cf. p. 119) can be useful to calm down any irritation.

Poor hygiene

The anus is sited quite close to the vulva. When combined with the fact that some small children might have a natural inclination to wipe forwards, meaning that any bacteria from faecal matter, such as *E. coli*, can be translocated (or moved) forwards to the vulval area, and it can become a site for irritation and infection.

Suggested treatments: If this has happens, follow the general advice below and look to support your child's immune system with medical mushrooms, some garlic in the diet and vitamin C (see the Immunity section, p. 124). Ensure that there is enough fibre in their diet. Also, do check for wiping forwards and if so, instruction on wiping front to back would be of great help in reducing recurrence. If an infection has occurred, probiotic powders could be sprinkled into the pants. If that doesn't shift it, it's worth going to see a qualified professional natural health practitioner for more targeted advice.

Pinworms

Very thin, white pinworms that look like uncooked egg noodles (though wriggly) are a parasitic worm infestation and can indeed inhabit the vagina, often transferred from the anus (which would be itchy) via eggs under fingernails transferred through scratching.[13] Not associated with hygiene issues, they can be seen in the vagina and cause a thin, colourless discharge with no smell. It can be difficult in some cases to convince a clinician that this is happening, which is unfortunate and unhelpful. Look for worms wriggling out of the faeces.[6] Support your child's immune system with medicinal mushrooms, some garlic in the diet and vitamin C.

Suggested treatments: If this is an issue for your child, adding raw carrot into their diet may be helpful as it is a vermifuge. It can be difficult to add in vermifuge or parasite killing herbs into their diets, due to the strong flavour. If that doesn't shift it, see a qualified professional natural health practitioner for more targeted advice.

Viruses

There are a whole host of viruses we can get tied up in being vigilant for, but touching on the major considerations, think about whether the child has had any full body viruses, such as varicella, measles or rubella, which may present on the skin over the whole body, and think about discharge. It's worth bearing in mind that, in children, vaginal discharge from viral infections appear as clear and watery. This is a helpful sign to look out for. *Herpes simplex* can present as vaginal discharge and be transmitted via vaginal labour or through possible sexual abuse.

Do not rule out molloscum contagiousm on the vulva too. Molluscum is caused by a viral infection of the skin, is very contagious, and appears mostly in children. It appears as small, round-shaped domes with dipped centres, and can be present on the vulva. They can last between 6–24 months if not treated and can resolve by themselves, but due to their contagious nature it may be preferable to seek treatment.

Suggested treatments: Look to support your child's immune system with medicinal mushrooms, some garlic in the diet and vitamin C (see the Immunity section, p. 124). Antiviral herbs such as St John's wort and/or lemon balm—infused in oil or ointments—may be applied topically. However, if that doesn't shift it after consistent treatment over the course of a couple of weeks, see a qualified professional natural health practitioner for more targeted advice.

Candida

As we will find out, *Candida* likes fuel to keep it growing and changing into its hyphal (more stubborn) form. In all cases, there is always a reason for its presence. In small children, damp nappies are the most likely cause and can be differentiated from other rashes as it is sore rather than itchy and because there are outlying spots around the main edge of the rash.[13] It is likely to be present mainly in the vulval area and possibly towards the inner thighs. If your child is past nappies, it is less likely to be *Candida* and it's always a good idea to get it tested before treating it with anti-fungal medicines, so we know we are using the correct and best treatment. If they have outgrown nappies and it proves to be *Candida*, you should always look at blood glucose (thinking diabetes) and sweet consumption as the fuel for *Candida*. Its presence warrants further investigation to rule out diabetes.

Suggested treatments: Look to support your child's immune system with medicinal mushrooms, some garlic in the diet and vitamin C (see the Immunity section, p. 124). You can also sprinkle probiotic powders onto their pants (note nothing should be placed into the vagina therapeutically in children). Calendula cream may also prove useful too. If these treatments don't shift it, see a qualified professional natural health practitioner for more targeted advice.

Bacterial

Often caused by microbes from the respiratory tract or skin (nose/ mouth to finger to vagina transmission, e.g. colds or impetigo), vaginal discharge in children with bacterial infections appears as a yellow or green colour. A smell may accompany it.

Suggested treatments: Look to support your child's immune system with medicinal mushrooms, some garlic in the diet and vitamin C (see the Immunity section, p. 124) and see a qualified professional natural health practitioner for more targeted advice if it persists.

Lichen sclerosis

This is an autoimmune, inflammatory, dermatological condition characterised by itchy white patches or areas that can be anywhere on the vulva or perineum. The skin can simply look paler in the affected areas. Although rare in children, it occurs most commonly in female children and middle-aged women. In female children, it appears as itching, soreness and blisters. It often resolves around puberty.[13] Ten per cent of those with lichen sclerosis are children.

Suggested treatments: Look to support your child's immune system with medicinal mushrooms, some garlic in the diet and vitamin C (see the Immunity section, p. 124) and see a qualified professional natural health practitioner for more targeted advice if it persists.

Other signs

Other signs could include birthmarks, attention-seeking behaviour, strawberry marks, and aphthous ulcers, which are ulcers associated with mucous membranes, such as you get in the mouth, but vaginally. These should clear up by themselves within 7–10 days.[13] A discharge containing mucous and pus or possibly even blood (past the initial eight weeks after birth)—could be a *Shigella* infection.

A thin, watery, foul-smelling discharge following an episode of diarrhoea could be an *E. Coli* infection.

It's worth bearing in mind that vaginal discharge from a child might be the only sign of sexual abuse in a child. This is worth being vigilant for and asking appropriate questions about, seeking further safeguarding and medical help as needed.

Some general advice for good intimate health for your female child

- Teach good hygiene to your child as soon as they are old enough to understand.
- Ensure the rectum is clean after defecation.
- Avoid constipation for your child—ensure good fibre levels and gently massage tummies if this is an issue.
- Teach them to wipe front to back.
- Avoid intimate soap use.
- Ensure the vulval area is totally dry after washing.
- Ensure the legs are properly apart when urinating to avoid moisture being trapped on the skin after urination.
- Avoid tight-fitting clothing.
- Wear natural fibre underwear—i.e. cotton or bamboo.
- Avoid wearing underwear to bed, if possible.
- Teach children not to put anything into their vaginas.

It's good to note that, in some cases, pharmaceutical medication may absolutely be needed here, but natural approaches can also be used to support their efficacy, improving overall outcomes for your child. If you don't start to see an improvement in any condition in your child within a few days to a week, don't let them suffer. Instead, seek help from a relevant health professional as soon as possible.

A word on consent

This may seem like a strange place to mention consent, but it is something worth bearing in mind. These days there is greater understanding and awareness of consent in all bodily matters, both sexual and non-sexual. This includes things such as parents asking rather than encouraging their children to hug or kiss visitors, and I think this is great on several levels—for one, it gives children greater autonomy over their bodies and their right to choose, and two it gives them a chance to practice saying no in a safe space. This is an empowering practice that, if handled well, promotes appropriate self-confidence. I think it goes hand in hand with teaching children the correct anatomical names for their body parts, about sex, masturbation and pleasure (when age-appropriate).

It is worth being mindful of this when taking children for intimate examinations at the GP. Obviously, it may be essential and the right thing to do for their care, but if they are old enough to understand what is going on, a conversation about what will happen during the exam and why might be useful. There is a lot of shame around intimate body parts in our culture. Normalising the body, pleasure, consent and what are considered 'embarrassing' health conditions from an early age might start to help break down the stigma and give our children the tools they need to empower themselves around consent and their sexual health. Imagine what changes that could bring about!

Adolescence and pre-menarch[11]

Back in the day, certainly when I was growing up (the 1980 and 90s—I know, ages ago!!), girls started their periods (a time known as the menarche) between 12 and 15, or maybe even earlier at 10 or 11, if they were especially 'early developers'. These days, the cold hard truth is that it's likely that some girls might start their periods as young as 8. While this is by no means the average—in fact they are statistical outliers—it's a factor to be aware of if we have daughters. It is likely that the age has come down by a few years due to endogenous hormones in our environment, food and water systems. This means we have man-made chemicals (exogenous—or, outside the body) which act like human sex hormones when they interact in or with the body.

These chemicals, in the main, come from the plastics humans use so prolifically. Even though, as a society we might recycle more, and as conscious consumers we may seek to use fewer plastics in our day-to-day, by-products from plastic breakdown leach into our food (tins that are lined with a thin film of plastic is one classic example). Another issue is bio-degradable (possibly compostable) plastic that we may herald as an answer to our planetary plastic woes. However, when this bio-degradable plastic breaks down, it breaks into microplastic particles that get into the food chain via the soil and our water systems (also think of the plastic straws that David Attenborough brought to our attention in his TV programmes).

Excess artificial oestrogens from the birth control pill pass out of the human body as urine ending up in the wider water system, joining the industrial pollution that still happens despite legislation. As a side note, you can get domestic water filtration systems using reverse osmosis technology that are able to filter out these exogenous oestrogens and provide cleaner water to drink. Exogenous oestrogens may also affect us during the fertile years and add to conditions in which excess oestrogen levels are implicated. Phew! These are some heavy and unsettling things to bear in mind. But, alas we must as it is the world we are given to live in and deal with.

As it is with the menopause, fluctuating hormonal changes that lead up to menarche happen over a period of time rather than switching on overnight. In many cases, once the first bleed has happened, there may be a time where periods are erratic while the hormone levels change and settle down. But what about the vaginal microbiome during this time? How do hormonal changes affect the vaginal tissues and environment?

Until recently, it was thought that up until menarche the vaginal microbiome stayed stable and similar to that of younger children as previously described. However, a recent study[14] which looked at this using 16S ribosomal RNA sampling, which is a method of identifying and classifying bacterial species, found that during the pre-menarche period the vaginal microbiome starts to be dominated by *Lactobacilli* colonies that change in response to hormonal fluctuations, as an adult woman's would. This happens over a relatively short period of time, much more quickly than other changes of puberty occur.

During this phase, oestrogen will also have the effect of thickening the labia minora and majora, and causing other sex organ and glandular changes we associate with puberty, such as the growth of pubic hair and breasts. It is at this time that girls may experience their first bouts of vulvovaginal candidiasis, aka thrush or other vulvovaginal irritation, due to these hormonal changes and impacts. A white, non-offensive smelling vaginal discharge (known as leukorrhea) may also occur and would be seen on the underpants. As long as this remains without a yeasty odour and is not accompanied by itch, it is nothing at all to worry about and simply a naturally occurring physiological discharge in response to hormone changes.

If itch or odour do occur, it is worth looking at getting some swabs done with the GP to see what is going on, and then looking at light-touch therapeutics to redress the balance, based on the diagnosis. The types of things that affect adult women of fertile age are now relevant for the prepubescent girl—but being a turbulent time it's not advisable to go in heavy-handed. Hormone levels can vary, which will have an impact on the experience of vaginal health and your approach should of course be directed by the severity of the issue, the symptoms experienced and the effect it is having on the quality of life. If a light-touch doesn't seem to have the desired effect, it may be time to seek the help of a professional, remembering the issues around explanation and consent. Conversation and communication are really important at this time to normalise vaginal health, making it a topic to which no shame or negativity is attached.

The biologically fertile years

Once the menstrual cycle has been established, at whatever age this occurs, the types of issues that might affect a woman in the fertile years of life will now be relevant for the adolescent girl. As already mentioned, it can take a number of months or years for her cycle to settle down, or her cycle could immediately become regular. Neither is right or wrong, and either way is entirely normal. During this time, it goes without saying that the process of sexual maturation is still being undertaken and she will not have finished physically developing yet.

A word on periods

While this book's primary focus isn't about hormonal health and periods specifically (there are plenty of other books out there covering this issue, a very good one in particular by this publisher), it's worth a page or two as sex hormones do impact greatly on the vaginal environment. It's a good idea to get a handle on what a 'normal' cycle is. A textbook definition of a cycle is one of 28 days in length (four weeks—the same amount of time as a lunar or moon cycle) and for many women this is what their cycle will look like for at least some part of their fertile life. However, for many it may be longer or it may be shorter, and it can change through life too. However it is for you is perfectly okay as long as it isn't causing you any physiological or health problems. There are no 'shoulds' around this. What is important to gather is that if you have roughly the same pattern and length to your cycle each month, that's ok. It's only not okay when you are experiencing issues that are causing you problems such as pain (contrary to popular belief, having a period is not meant to hurt), emotional disturbance, very heavy bleeding etc. If you notice something like this, go have a chat with your herbalist.

A word about the term 'fertile years' or 'fertile life'. I've really thought about whether to use these terms. I am using them to refer to biological processes, but I am aware that it might feel exclusionary, indicating that if you have passed through menopause, or have a premature or medically induced menopause, there is an inference that you are no longer a fertile, creative being—'fertile' here referring to the act of creation and creativity. On the contrary, the wisdom and confidence women in this stage of life are imbued with allows for some of their most creative work, and should be celebrated. I use 'fertile' in the sense of biologically being able to conceive another human. Onwards ...

During the biologically fertile years there are a set of specific conditions and issues that may play out for a woman. This is due not only to the nature of the vaginal environment as delicately controlled by the hormones, but also the types of activities that it is normal to engage in: sex, menstruation and the use of menstrual products, diet, exercise.

Many women may go through this time in their life without being plagued by any particular issues and some will not be so lucky. For example, did you know that over 70% of all women will experience thrush (also known as vaginal candidiasis) at least once in their life? No big deal, you might think. But did you know that between 5 and 9% of these women will go on to experience it recurrently? That's counted as at least four times a year, often more.

Did you also know that it is possible for you to have two or more intimate infections at the same time, or switch between two, as the vaginal microbiome swings one way and then the other? Thrush and bacterial vaginosis can, but thankfully not always, work like this.

The thing is, once you get into a situation where intimate dysbiosis becomes entrenched it can be hard to break out of it—just look at all the posts in the Facebook groups dedicated to overcoming conditions such as thrush and bacterial vaginosis. There are literally thousands of women there. Be thankful if this is not you, but know what to do if it is.

No one was listening to me, no one was taking me seriously. It took me 12 years to get an endometriosis diagnosis. Painful, vomit-inducing periods, thrush, migraines, tiredness, low moods; I had no idea that they were all related. I went to the doctors, time after time all they wanted to offer me was hormonal pills.

Stop.

Listen.

Listen to your body.

You know your body.

You are your body.

Empower yourself in a world that is so disempowering.

I was lucky. I found someone to guide me on my journey, who listened to my body, who listened to nature. Who listened to me. It took me 12 years of screaming into closed doors and she gave me the key. She reflected back to me what my body had been trying to tell me for years. She helped me to tune in to my body and trust what I heard, felt, knew.

—Vicki

pH and testing

When we talked about the vaginal microbiome we spoke about vaginal pH. The pH is a scale from 0 to 14 that defines how acidic or basic (chemistry term for alkaline) a water-based solution is. What it actually measures is the concentration of hydrogen ions—the higher the concentration, the more acidic the solution is. pH 7 is classed as neutral, neither acidic nor alkaline. The pH of the epidermis (human skin) is around 5.5—so on the acid side of things, and this is part of an innate protection against infection called the acid mantle. If you recall, vaginal pH sits at around 3.8–4.5. That's pretty acidic, somewhere in the range of orange juice and acid rain (think bleached knickers).

The reason we want it to be acidic, and why the *Lactobacilli* work in harmony with the body to create it thus is so that it keeps the 'bad', and yet commonly present, bacteria and yeast under control and at bay. To be clear, many of the bacteria and fungi that cause the issues we are about to dive deep into (that's a nice image isn't it?!) are found quite naturally and normally in the vagina. This means they are known as commensal microbes, and if they are kept in their place (by the environmental conditions down there), they don't cause any issues.

None of these conditions are caused by being dirty, although good hygiene practices can definitely help! Many of the bacterial types that cause the conditions below thrive in an alkaline environment and can cause the vaginal environment to move away from its happy acidic habitat. Things that promote a more alkaline environment, such as semen (yes, semen is an alkaline substance) can cause an overgrowth of these bacteria. It's a chicken-and-egg situation.

The type of yeast that can cause thrush, *Candida*, however, does like an acid environment too. If you have got something going on vaginally (and don't assume it's thrush because it's uncomfortable), one of the basic tests you can do for yourself to work out the likelihood of what you have is a pH test. You can buy one over the counter in pharmacies, under a well-known brand name, or you can go onto a well-known e-commerce site and buy yourself some pH test strips. Make sure they are the stiff-type strips and not litmus paper. When your symptoms are at their worst, get some of the discharge onto one of the strips and test it.

Above 4.5 and you might be looking at a bacterial imbalance, rather than a yeast. It puts some power in your hands and is useful to tell me if you come to work with me clinically. I would also recommend you have a swab from the GP to then get a clearer idea of exactly what microbe is causing the issue. Even if you think you've had the symptoms before and you think you know what is going on.

Swabs

Ah, the delight of swabs (and pap smear tests—they fall into this category of delight too—more about those later!). They've really managed to create a situation so unpleasant and undignified but yet so vital for the health of women, that it is really off-putting to almost all, while being such a vital part of our medical- and self-care. (Another serving of cognitive dissonance surrounding vaginas anyone?!)

I always recommend that the clients I work with go and get a swab from their GP if they haven't done so before they've come to see me, because it is with a swab that we start to see a glimpse into what is going on in the microbial community of the vagina. We can then proceed with the correct types of treatment. Nothing worse than thinking you have one thing, attempting to treat it but wondering why it's not working. We also need to be sure that nothing more sinister, i.e. damaging, is going on.

So, before trying to treat anything, we need to know what we are working with, and swabs are one way to do this. The technical name for these swabs is a high vaginal swab or wet mount. A small cotton-tipped swab is inserted into the vagina to collect a sample of the microbiome, which is then sent to the histology department at your local hospital to be cultured (getting what is there to grow further for easier identification) and then identified and counted under a microscope. The results are then sent back to the GP.

Swabbing can be really handy and certainly gives us a more advanced picture than we get with pH testing alone, but it relies on whatever is there to be cultured to the point that it can be identified and counted. It's worth noting that reporting standards differ from area to area, and you may not receive a precise picture of the species present.

There are private tests coming onto the market now utilising quantitative real-time PCR testing to analyse the DNA of the microbes that make up the vaginal microbiome. These can be done at home, are minimally invasive and don't rely on culture and microscopy. They give a clearer picture, but are expensive and shouldn't be done without working with an experienced clinician who can interpret and explain the results, as they can be quite confusing. However, it's worth knowing about them in case you really need to get to the bottom of a situation that isn't making sense.

Common conditions during the fertile years

Bacterial vaginosis

What is it: Bacterial vaginosis, or 'BV' for those 'lucky' enough to be in the know, is characterised by an overgrowth of mostly anaerobic bacteria. These are bacteria that thrive in an oxygen-poor environment, such as a vagina might present. The primary culprits are *Gardnerella vaginalis*, *Atopobium vaginae* and *Prevotella* spp. (spp. is short for 'species' and is often used when describing a genera of bacteria or plants, i.e. a few species in the same family—you'll find it several times throughout this book). However, several other bacteria species can be associated with a BV type state. These include *Mobiluncus* spp., *Megasphaera 1* and 2 and

BVAB2. These bacteria can exist happily side by side in the vagina next to *Lactobacilli* and cause no problem, and it is quite normal to find them in the vaginal microbiome, but it is when conditions ideal for these bacteria to proliferate occur that they overgrow and become problematic. When they do overgrow to dominate the vaginal space, they cause the environment to become more alkaline at a pH of 5 or higher. This in turn makes it difficult for the *Lactobacilli* to survive and keep everything functioning well in the environment.

What symptoms are likely: The most common symptoms are a thin, watery clear to greyish discharge that seems to 'gush' out when you move or do anything that changes the internal pressure in your body and involves core muscle movement, like coughing, flatulence or burping. In some cases this discharge can have a yellowish to green colour, but in all cases it is characterised by its thin, watery nature.

Another tell-tale symptom is a fishy, metallic or unpleasant smelling discharge. This classic smell is caused by the by-products of the bacterium, and can be tested for in the discharge by your health care provider carrying out a 'whiff test' (where Potassium Hydroxide (KOH) is added to the discharge to test for the presence of amines).

What else it could be: Most often confused with thrush, the prevalence of BV is similar to thrush in the female population, but can be differentiated by the type of discharge, smell, presence of itch, the presence of clue cells (specific to BV) on testing, and the pH value. With thrush the pH can be in the normal acid range of 3.8–4.5—with BV it is often higher than this, being more alkaline. The discharge with thrush can be white and cottage cheese-like, with a yeasty smell (think fresh bread), and often accompanied by an itch. If you're not sure, a pH test can help differentiate.

It is also possible to get thrush at the same time as BV and vice versa, or BV followed by thrush, followed again by BV if you are unlucky. If this is going on, see a specialist. BV can also present similarly to trichomoniasis, which is caused by a parasite that can be passed through sexual contact, creating an unpleasant smell and a yellow-green discharge. However, this discharge is frothy. If there is any doubt, always go to your GP for a swab test.

More about it: The Vaginosis part of the name means that it is considered, in general, a non-inflammatory condition. Contrast this with aerobic vaginitis further on, where the term vaginitis indicates that it is an inflammatory condition.

In conventional medicine, a go-to 'standard' treatment would be a course of the antibiotic Metronidazole. BV that has produced a biofilm will often be resistant to this treatment. Biofilms are when a bacterial colony, in this case 'bad bacterium', have created their own mucous matrices, which are an ideal environment for them and makes it harder for therapeutics to penetrate treat the area. One of the bacterium that is responsible for BV, *Atopobium vaginae* is also resistant to Metronidazole. If you take Metronidazole and this does not clear it consider that it could be for one or both of these two reasons.

Another, newer, treatment that is now being prescribed for BV is a vaginal gel that contains lactic acid and glycogen. It can be bought over the counter without a prescription and works by encouraging the growth and maintenance of a *Lactobacilli* rich environment, which will keep the 'bad' guys in check. This is a good aim for treatment and has clinical evidence to back it up (there are several brands on the market).

How we get it: The first thing to state is that although it is caused by bacteria, having BV does not mean that you are 'dirty' or 'unclean'. Overgrowth of the bacteria responsible is due to a change in the environment, meaning that the *Lactobacilli* are no longer dominant. Things such as hormone levels, antibiotics, and the presence of semen, menstrual blood, douching or alkaline lubricants can all be causes in the first instance, and it is important to work out the cause at the same time as treatment to try and prevent recurrence. In some cases, as mentioned above, BV can become stubborn or reoccur and may require a different approach to the standard treatment.

Approaches and aims: In many cases a short course of antibiotics might be able to clear it up, without setting off a thrush outbreak— less likely if you don't have a history of thrush. If it doesn't (and some microbes are resistant to the antibiotics regularly prescribed for BV), or you want to steer clear of antibiotics, the vaginal gels are a good option, along with a course of probiotics that contain *L. rhamnosus* and *L. gasseri*. There is research that has shown that these can translocate from the gut to support the microbiome via the faecal-vagina route.

The aims of any approach here are to support the reformation of a healthy, *Lactobacilli* rich microbiome. If you are experiencing BV that simply won't budge, it's recurrent, or mixed in with thrush, then see a qualified registered complementary health practitioner who specialises in vaginal health for further strategies and treatment.

It's also worth noting that studies have shown that smoking is a risk factor for BV, as smoking has been linked to a lower population of beneficial *Lactobacillus* types of bacteria in their vaginal microbiomes than non-smokers.[36] If this is going on for you and you are a smoker it might be another reason to rethink quitting.

Suggested treatments: Therapeutics in the Antimicrobial (p. 155) and pH Modulation sections (p. 153) would be specific here.

Cautions: It's worth being on top of BV because its presence can be linked with an increased risk of acquiring STDs and an increased risk for miscarriage or pre-term birth.

Thrush

What is it: Thrush is the opportunistic overgrowth of yeast cells in the vaginal space. The most likely cause of thrush is the *Candida* spp. of yeasts, and the most common of these is *Candida albicans*. This species causes between 70–90% of all cases of thrush.

These *Candida* spp. can live in bud form commensally (alongside) with a happy, healthy vaginal microbiome without causing any issues, and this is the case for up to 70% of all women. It is only when conditions occur that are favourable for the overgrowth of the yeasts that a problem is likely to arise. As they grow, the buds develop into a hyphal form of the yeast, which then can adhere to and 'burrow' into the mucosal tissue that lines the vagina, taking up a more aggressive residence. This can make it much more difficult to clear it and is one of the reasons some women have stubborn cases.

Another reason some women find difficulty in clearing it is due to the fact in 5–18% of cases, recurrent thrush is caused by a different species of *Candida*, *Candida glabrata*, which is not affected by the regular medication that a GP can prescribe or can be bought over the counter.

Unlike BV, chronic or recurrent thrush is unlikely to change vaginal pH and is perfectly happy growing in a more acidic environment, although a change may be detected in an acute case. The correct medical name for thrush is vulvovaginal candidiasis (VVC).

What symptoms are likely: The most common symptoms are itch, burning and sometimes pain, a white discharge that can be cottage cheesy in appearance and smell yeasty. These can be experienced either on the vulva, in the vagina or both. Thrush can also cause inflammation and there is likely to be redness in the areas affected.

What else it could be: As mentioned above, it's most often confused with BV and it is worth getting a test to make 100% sure of what you are dealing with. The confusion seems to be most often caused by the fact that both have discharge and are not considered STIs (although they can be transferred sexually). However, there is a great difference in the appearance and quality of the discharge that both create. If it's a white, chunky discharge, that can appear slightly yellowy on toilet paper, it's more likely to be thrush. Also, see if there is a fishy or unpleasant odour: thrush will only have a yeasty/bready type smell.

One other, much less likely condition that it can be confused with is cytolytic vaginosis, which is outlined below. This also has a white discharge but is characterised by a different microbiome profile type. A swab can help determine if *Candida* spp. is the cause!

More about it: Over 70% of women globally will suffer from thrush at least once in their lifetime. Most of these cases will be isolated incidents with a clear, or at least suspected, cause, and classic symptoms which respond to treatment and then resolve. These cases are called acute cases because there are marked symptoms with a sudden onset, cause, and in the case of thrush, a defined resolution.

However, for 5–9% of those women listed above, they go on to have recurrent outbreaks of thrush. Recurrent thrush (RVVC) is defined as having thrush four or more times in a 12-month period. It is likely that something is going on to cause this recurrence, such as the stubborn types mentioned above or an incident for the individual that is making them susceptible, outlined below.

For a case to be classed as recurrent there is a defined period in which the flare-up happens and then it appears to resolve (often during or around the menses, and perhaps for a time after that) and then returns again.

It is classed as a chronic (CVVC) case when there is no break or let up between flare-ups and it is always present in the background, occasionally coming to the foreground.

People who tend towards the chronic or recurrent forms may be more likely to suffer from allergic conditions such as allergic rhinitis, asthma or eczema (although this is not always the case), and there is less likely to be a change in the microbiome. The cell walls of the *Candida* spp. contain elements that mean they can 'hide' and not be adequately detected by the immune system in many cases.

How we get it: For acute one-off cases, an incident such as taking antibiotics might create just the right conditions (a temporary reduction in the vaginal *Lactobacilli* because they have been killed off by the antibiotics) for an overgrowth. For many women, once it is resolved that's the last they need to think of it. However, this may set up the optimal conditions for a recurrent or chronic pattern to form. In order for this to occur, certain other situations will likely be present in the body, which can include, but are not limited to, a weakened immune system, hormone imbalance, poorly controlled blood sugar levels, digestion issues and allergic tendencies. These may not be causing visible issues in other areas of the body (though they might) and may be subclinical—just enough to cause a disturbance.

Some other factors that contribute to opportunistic growth of *Candida* spp. include atopic allergy; local pH changes; warm, wet environments that do not get a chance to dry out; intimate washing with soaps; fabric washing agents; toilet paper; certain hobbies such as cycling or rowing; and the hygiene and condition of sex aids and toys. Risk factors including taking oestrogen medications such as the oral contraceptive pill or HRT, or pregnancy.

Approaches and aims: Aims for treating this condition are to reduce itch, pain and inflammation to give you some relief, and restoring a healthy microbiome, which will help keep the yeasts in their place. Anti-fungal herbs have their place in doing this, possibly in the form of pessaries, and taken orally so that the whole body can absorb them. Topical anti-inflammatory herbs such as chamomile, green tea and calendula can be used as cooling washes, and aloe vera gel may provide symptomatic relief (if it's driving you crazy, putting the tube of gel in the fridge for a while first may help to bring even more relief)!

If it is a simple case of acute *Candida albicans* (confirmed by swab), then a cream pessary by a well-known pharmaceutical brand might clear it in one go. In the more chronic or recurrent types of thrush it is important to protect the delicate tissue of the vulva and vagina through minimising sexual interaction, scratching and lubrication. Visit a qualified, registered complementary healthcare professional that specialises in vaginal health to get to the root cause of the situation, where lifestyle and dietary interventions will often make up part of any plan which can help with the prevention of future flare-ups.

It's also very worthwhile noting anything that seems to make it better or worse, and then avoiding the things that make it worse. This can include foods, underwear fabrics, washing powders, certain clothing types, certain sexual acts, certain washing habits, types of toilet paper ... When you have a flare-up the list of what makes it worse could feel endless (see Part Five for some ideas).

Suggested treatments: Therapeutics in the Mucous membrane integrity (p. 135) and Anti-fungal sections (p. 161) and old man's beard in the Antimicrobial section (p. 155) would be specific here. Abdominal massage (cf. p. 114) would also be supportive.

Cautions: Thrush is an inflammatory condition, which may also involve tissue damage due to hyphae infiltration, and as such leaves the vaginal mucosa at risk of damage in the form of micro tears and from scratching due to the itch. This damage makes it much more likely for other opportunistic bacteria, including sexually transmitted infections (STIs) to have a chance to take hold in this space, so it is worth being mindful of this if you are suffering a flare-up.

Don't

It's the prickling feeling, between your legs.

You don't want to go out. Thinking about going out makes you crawl.

You've got to go out.

Let me settle, but you can't. Let. Me. Settle. You can't settle.

Your pants feel wet and awkward. You pack prickly cottage cheese in the folds.

Has it soaked through your trousers?
No, don't be silly. Don't be silly. Feel to check. Don't touch.

Your hair and fabrics irritate the skin. Your vulva is on fire.

A thigh gap would actually have a use right now.

Instead, try to walk so your thighs don't touch. Just look normal. Don't touch.

A friend is talking to you. Concentrate. On their words.

You want to air out, stop wet sore skin rubbing   on   wet
sore skin   on sore wet skin, on wet

                    You feel a bit light headed.

                S t r e t c h i n g

Leggings make you burn

                    are hysterical in jeans.

Concentrate on their words.
Just look normal.
Don't touch.

You can't work out if you need to pee. Do you?
It's the feeling of wanting to wipe, yes, to attend to the area.
But bog roll irritates, scrapes at the skin. Bright red skin. Don't
touch.

just to be cool and dry and soothed. Attend to the area.

Get home.

Get naked. Get dry. And alone
In private. You feel anxious while you're out. Prickly.

Quick, look. Mirror in your hands.
The skin looks like nappy rash. It shocks you to see it. Don't.

Got to get home. Don't go out.

But
it's not because you're dirty. Dirt has nothing to do with it.

You are clean. But you feel dirty.

don't do dirty.
Don't scratch.

DON'T scratch ...
Don't think about it.
Don't even think about it.
Don't

~ Skin weeps ~

get it out of me ...

                just

            don't

                                —Kathie

Cytolytic vaginosis

What is it: Nowhere near as prevalent as thrush, it's likely that you haven't heard about cytolytic vaginosis (CV) before. Also known as *Lactobacillus* overgrowth syndrome, it is diagnosed by the absence of pathogenic bacteria in the vaginal environment, but a marked and unusual increase in the 'good' *Lactobacillus* spp. of bacteria. Being a vaginosis rather than a vaginitis, it is characterised by a lack of inflammation.

What symptoms are likely: A white creamy discharge, itchiness, discomfort, and pain during sex and urination are the most likely symptoms. Some people may also report that the discharge tastes acidic if ingested and if any discharge comes into contact with a cut it might cause irritation. In some cases these symptoms increase at and following mid-cycle ovulation. With symptoms so similar to thrush it's no surprise that it is often misdiagnosed!

What else it could be: As the symptoms are so similar to thrush, please go and have a swab taken at the GP to see what they can culture. Many countries and regions do not have a specific test for it and so the absence of *Candida* spp. and a worsening of symptoms on taking probiotics might be your best indication! Other possibilities include BV, trichomoniasis and aerobic vaginitis. A home pH test will indicate a lower pH reading than the normal range of 3.8–4.5 because in CV the environment becomes more acidic than it should!

More about it: Recent research has shown that *L. crispatus* (the *Lactobacilli* normally associated with vaginal health and the highest producer of lactic acid) might be the main microbe associated with CV. If there is too much of this and an absence of any anaerobic bacteria—such as those associated with BV—then cytolytic vaginosis may occur.

How we get it: The root cause is unclear but it might be a 'rebound' after restoring an unbalanced vaginal environment with 'healthy' *Lactobacilli*. There might also be a history of antibiotics, hormone imbalance, douching, poorly regulated blood sugar levels and diabetes.

Approaches and aims: The aim here is to reduce the number of *Lactobacilli* and restore the correct pH range. Bearing in mind that *Lactobacilli* are bacteria, the way conventional medicine may deal with it is via antibiotics. A holistic approach will look to decrease the symptoms and *Lactobacilli* number with Bi-carb sitz baths while supporting the body to provide the correct environment for a healthy microbiome. That environment would be one that is slightly more diverse than it has become with this condition and more alkaline. It can be a lengthy and challenging process and for that reason it would be advisable to work with a qualified, registered complementary health practitioner that specialises in vaginal health.

Suggested treatments: Therapeutics in the pH modulation section (p. 153) would be specific here.

Cautions: Be aware that antibiotic treatment may 'kill off' too many of the good bacteria, tipping the balance the other way and potentially allowing any lurking *Candida* spp. or bacteria that have translocated from the rectum to flourish. Any antibiotics may also impact on your digestive microbiome too!

Aerobic vaginitis

What is it: Aerobic vaginitis, or AV, is a disruption of the vaginal microbiome by aerobic (oxygen-loving) bacteria, such as Group B *Streptococcus*, *Enterococcus faecalis*, *E. Coli* and *S. aureus*, causing amongst other things, inflammation (note that BV, caused by anaerobic bacteria, doesn't particularly create inflammation).

What symptoms are likely: Often one of the most common symptoms is burning around the vaginal opening, yellow to yellow-green discharge, visible reddening of the skin, itchiness, burning, pain on swimming or bathing and possible lesions and bleeding. There may also be an unpleasant odour that tests as negative on whiff testing (described under the Bacterial vaginosis section). On a home pH test the pH will be above 4.5 but less than 6.

It is diagnosed conclusively by microscopy and culture from a swab test.

What else it could be: Because of the similar presentation of discharge to trichomoniasis, as well as thrush and BV, testing should be undertaken to get a clear diagnosis. Testing in this case is important to rule out infection of the cervix or lining of the womb.

More about it: It is possible to get AV at the same time as a *Candida* overgrowth which will complicate the picture and treatment. As AV affects the integrity of the vaginal tissues, sex may be painful.

Chronic AV, aka desquamative inflammatory vaginitis (DIV), which *E. Coli* or *Strep B.* are primarily responsible for causing, can become quite extreme if left untreated or misdiagnosed and can cause great amounts of vaginal discharge and pain. Cervical changes at the cellular level can also be observed, so if you suspect this, press for correct diagnosis.

How we get it: Many of the bacteria associated with AV are bacteria that also live in the intestinal tract. It is possible that translocation (movement of bacteria in this case from one area to another, through hygiene practices) is responsible for the development of this condition. There may also be a link to a vitamin D deficiency, Lichen planus (see below), hormone imbalance and immune issues.

Approaches and aims: The aims and approaches here are really to regain *Lactobacilli* dominance, reduce the aerobic bacteria, and help maintain the tissue coherence of the vaginal tissues. Antimicrobial herbs and probiotics definitely form part of the healing picture and may be used as pessaries. Supplementing with vitamin D may prove useful. This shouldn't be one of the things that you try to treat at home alone. You need the support of a healthcare professional and this may be in the form of both conventional medicine and a qualified, registered complementary health care professional specialising in vaginal health.

Suggested treatments: Therapeutics in the Mucous membrane integrity (p. 135), Antimicrobial (p. 155) sections and probiotics as pessaries (cf. p. 154) would be specific here.

Cautions: Due to its link with cervical changes and complications in pregnancy and conception, the misdiagnosis and mismanagement of AV can lead to a number of complications such as pelvic inflamma-tory disease, infertility, miscarriage, pre-term delivery and cervical wall changes. It is worth noting that in the UK if you are at high risk of or symptomatic for AV in pregnancy, you are screened for it. I know this sounds scary and I haven't included it here to freak you out, but to be clear that if you suspect AV and you're diagnosed with something else which does not respond to treatment, you need to press for the correct diagnosis.

Mollicutes

What is it: Mollicutes are bacteria that have no cell walls. They are passed on by sexual contact and during vaginal birth. There are two main genera involved in vaginal and cervical versions, known as *Myco-plasma* and *Ureaplasma*. *Ureaplasmas* makes up 40–80% of all cases of mollicutes while two species of *Mycoplasma* cover the rest—*M. hominis* makes up 20–50% of cases, and *M. genitalium* makes up to 5% of cases and is considered an STI. In many cases they can exist in an otherwise healthy vaginal microbiome causing no symptoms—often conventional medicine will not think that they are worthy of treatment unless you are trying to conceive.

What symptoms are likely: Although it is often without symptoms, a thick white, otherwise non-offensive discharge is common, with pos-sible bleeding mid-month and after sex. It might also cause pain on passing urine. In very acute cases it can cause pelvic pain.

What else it could be: It's important to get tested to rule out other STIs.

More about it: *Ureaplasma* and *M. hominis* have both been associated with premature birth, so if you are trying to get pregnant it's important to seek diagnosis and treatment beforehand. Diagnosis is via vaginal swab.

How we get it: Not uncommon in childhood because it can be passed from the mother to baby via vaginal delivery, after puberty the main route of transmission is through sexual intercourse.

Approaches and aims: As previously stated, the conventional approach will not seek to clear mollicutes infection, unless trying to conceive. This may be in part because these microbes now have a high level of resistance to antibiotics. If you are treated for *Mycoplasma* or *Ureaplasma*, its worth getting a re-test at three months post-treatment to check to see if it has indeed cleared!

However, with a complementary approach there are many other things that can be done. As in all cases with vaginal health, encouraging a healthy vaginal environment of *Lactobacilli* and pH is important—as is clearing the mollicute microbes with antimicrobial herbs. If there is any difficulty in treatment (i.e. the mollicutes are resisting treatment), we may need to look at strategies that clear a biofilm. We must also support the immune system to do its job effectively. As part of any treatment approach, it is wise to also modify normal sexual behaviours to avoid contact with any mollicutes that your partner may be carrying, which could re-infect you. It would be wise to treat your partner/s during this time also.

Suggested Treatments: Therapeutics in the Antimicrobial section (p. 155), as well as those in the Mucous membrane integrity section (p. 135) and probiotics as pessaries (cf. p. 154) would be specific here.

Cautions: This set of microbes are implicated in miscarriage and premature birth so it is important to clear them if detected, before trying to conceive. Once clear, it's important not to have intercourse with a partner until 14 days after they are tested and cleared following treatment themselves, or test as negative if they haven't been treated. Otherwise, you could become reinfected again!

Lichen sclerosus

What is it: Lichen sclerosus is a chronic autoimmune condition that affects the vulval tissues and the skin around the anus. White blood cells, which are a component of the immune system and the blood accumulate in the vulval tissues and release inflammatory chemicals into the area. Over time the skin loses its pigmentation and flexibility and becomes waxy or crinkled. This means that it can tear or crack easily, and penetrative intercourse can become very painful and difficult due to the narrowing of the opening of the vagina.

What symptoms are likely: In addition to the above, the labia can become atrophied and stuck together, and the clitoral hood (prepuce) can become scarred, covering the clitoris in scar tissue. Vulvar itching, burning and pain may also occur, alongside tearing of the skin and reduced clitoral sensation or a feeling of pressure on the clitoris.

What else it could be: Lichen planus (see below).

More about it: The earliest signs of LS can be fragile skin tearing and blistering. It can cause hyperpigmentation as well. Half of the cases tend to be in menopausal women, but up to 10% can be in female children, with the remaining 40% being women of fertile age.

How we get it: LS seems to be of unknown cause, but with autoimmune disorders there is some form of immune dysregulation causing the immune system to attack 'self', rather than 'other'.

Approaches and aims: This is a great opportunity where natural health can support any pharmaceutical intervention. I would recommend having allopathic support as well as a more natural approach in the management of LS, and biopsy may be offered. Look to support the healthy functioning of the immune system with medicinal mushrooms, marigold teas and echinacea, as well as looking to reduce the inflammatory load in the body via diet and anti-inflammatory herbs. Soothing anti-inflammatory creams with plantain or marshmallow root may also provide some relief to epithelial tissue. Also, consider mucosal membrane support with essential fatty acids and sea buckthorn oil, taken internally. Sitz baths may also prove useful for a feeling of relief. Consider using oat, marigold and chamomile here. If it doesn't improve after trying to treat it yourself, please seek the advice of a qualified medical herbalist.

Suggested treatments: Therapeutics in the Immunity (p. 124), Anti-inflammatory (p. 119), Mucous membrane integrity (p. 135) and Nervines (p. 140) sections would be specific here.

Cautions: Due to chronic inflammation, there is statistically a 5% risk that LS can turn to cancer. In conventional treatment, potent topical steroids are used on the area in a way that may cause skin thinning. There are careful protocols in place to try and reduce the incidence of this.

Lichen planus

What is it: Lichen planus (LP) is another chronic autoimmune skin disease that may appear in other parts of the body—25% of cases affect the vulva or vagina. Unlike LS, LP can affect the vagina as well as the vulva, meaning that both areas can be scarred. In LP the mucosa develops plaques and erosions rather than the waxy appearance of LS, and these areas of erosion can have a lacy-edged appearance known as Wickham's Stria.[10]

What symptoms are likely: Itchy plaques and lesions with flat surfaces which are about 2–4 mm in diameter. These lesions can be on other parts of the body as well as the vulva and vagina and are violet in colour. New lesions can develop at the site of tissue trauma caused by activities such as scratching, and in the later stages can coalesce together. They can also change over time in colour and texture.

What else it could be: Lichen sclerosis (see above). Also, watch out for lupus and secondary syphilis, which can present in a similar fashion. Diagnosis is given by appearance rather than swabbing, and a biopsy may be needed to confirm.

More about it: Plaques are also found in the mucosal membranes of the mouth about 50% of the time, and also may appear in the soft folds of major joints such as the elbow and knee. In 10% of cases, nails and nail beds can also be involved. Cases of LP can be resolved without intervention if the trigger, such as an LP-causing drug, mentioned below, is stopped. It can reoccur again if the trigger is reintroduced.[11] It may also be symptomless.

How we get it: Lichen planus is thought to have a genetic component, although it has been noted that certain drugs (B-blockers, NSAIDs, ACE inhibitors, *Sulphonylureas*, antimalarial agents, penicillamine, and thiazides) can induce LP, so check if you are taking any of these and ask for a review from the prescribing clinician. It is also possible that it is associated with hepatitis C induced liver insufficiency.[15]

Approaches and aims: Natural medicine can play its role alongside pharmaceutical intervention, by supporting the healthy functioning of the immune system with medicinal mushrooms, marigold tea and echinacea, as well as reducing the inflammatory load in the body via diet and anti-inflammatory herbs. Soothing anti-inflammatory creams with plantain or marshmallow root may also provide some relief to epithelial tissue. Consider mucosal membrane support with essential fatty acids and sea buckthorn oil, taken orally. Sitz baths may also prove useful for a feeling of relief. Consider using oat, marigold and chamomile here. If it doesn't improve after trying to treat it yourself, please seek the advice of a qualified medical herbalist.

Suggested treatments: Therapeutics in the Immunity (p. 124), Anti-inflammatory (p. 119), Mucous membrane integrity (p. 135) and Nervines (p. 140) sections would be specific here.

Cautions: In a conventional approach, if the LP is on multiple sites on the body, topical treatment can be impractical. It is a systemic condition, rather than just affecting the vagina and vulva.

Cystic glands

The two sets of glands that sit inside the vestibule of the vulva—Bartholin's glands and the Skene's glands can become blocked, creating swollen cysts. Sometimes they form without causing symptoms and don't require treatment. However, if symptoms occur such as interference with intercourse and walking, pain, fever and redness (in the case of the Bartholin's cysts), and obstruction of the flow of urine or UTIs (in the case of Skene's gland cysts), they may require drainage.

It is important to understand that any of the conditions above can cause your vulva and vagina to become more sensitised to pain or discomfort. This is especially true if you are suffering from recurring infections, as you can begin to be on the lookout for any feeling that may indicate the problem is about to return. Not only are your tissues feeling primed to sense anything untoward happening, but your mind is also on the lookout too. As we discussed in Part Two—where we looked at the anatomy and physiology of the vulva and vagina—this whole area has a rich supply of nerves, which not only delivers pleasure but, if sensitised, can also dish out the pain.

The mind–body relationship is a complex one, and such a richly innervated and sensual area will have a lot of feedback between the body and mind, and mind and body back to the intimate areas again. This means emotions can impact the vulva and vagina and vice versa. I see this time and time again in clinical practice. More on this a little later—but bear in mind the concept while we cover the next couple of conditions.

Suggested treatments: Therapeutics in the Immunity (p. 124) and Anti-inflammatory (p. 119) sections would be supportive here.

Vulvodynia, vestibulodynia, clitoridynia and pain

What is it: A diagnosis of any of these means that you are suffering pain in your vulva, vestibule or clitoris, and the medical establishment can't find a cause for it. That doesn't mean that there isn't a cause; it's just that the correct cause hasn't been identified and could be different for each person. For example, an overly tight pelvic floor could cause nerve pain. *Dynia* literally means pain in Ancient Greek. Pain is detected and transmitted to the brain when the nerve cells in the area perceive damage in some respect. The cause can be varied, but there is *always* a cause. It can even be caused by a sensitisation of the nerves in the area that are 'set off' by regular everyday activities like walking, touching, or without any stimuli at all!

What symptoms are likely: Burning, searing or throbbing pain in the area affected. It has been described as feeling as though there are razor blades, knives or a lit cigarette lighter in your vagina. It can be agonising and very disruptive to someone's life.

What else it could be: Vaginismus, or vaginitis.

More about it: Research from 2003 has shown that up to a third of all women that experience vulval pain never seek help for it,[10] which is a terrible fact in itself and we should wonder why help is never sought. Vulvodynia is a generalised term, meaning that the pain that you suffer is throughout your vulva and vestibule areas. vestibulodynia (or provoked vestobulodynia) is the most common cause of sexual pain and it is estimated that up to 16% of women have it,[8] being triggered by contact. Clitorodynia can sometimes be caused by nerve pain to the clitoris following a herpes infection.[8]

How we get it: There doesn't seem to be one single cause of any of these painful conditions, although they sometimes appear after using vaginal medication of one sort or another. For some, there might be no identifiable trigger, while for others it can occur from the first time they use a tampon. It appears that whatever is triggering this nerve pain, it's a neurological condition resulting from dysfunctional nerve fibres that overreact to normal stimuli and don't switch off once the stimuli ends. This is referred to as 'pain windup'. The overactive nerves feed into the dorsal horn of the spinal cord, which acts as a gate keeper to determine which pain impulses get transmitted to the brain, how strongly they are transmitted and which endogenous (body-generated) pain-receiving chemicals, such as endorphins, get released.[8]

Women who suffer from this are more likely to suffer from other chronic pain conditions too, such as interstitial cystitis and fibromyalgia. This situation is referred to as complex regional pain syndrome (CRPS). One theory as to why it occurs is that it is caused by damage to the pudendal nerve—even minor damage through a fall, childbirth or pressure from sitting on a bike seat may cause it. Because nerve damage cannot be seen, many doctors do not appreciate that this kind of pain is not imagined.

In addition, provoked vestibulodynia has been linked to taking the oral contraceptive pill, plus there's an idea that there might be an over-abundance of nerve endings in the vestibule of the individual concerned.

Approaches and aims: To help reduce this kind of nerve pain we need to get a clearer understanding of whether there is a tightened pelvic floor (a female pelvic physiotherapist can help determine this) and whether there are any inflammation or triggers, such as taking the pill. Once this has been determined, appropriate remedial action can be taken.

Avoid fabrics that might irritate (organic cotton or bamboo might be good options) and wash only with water. If able to be sexually active, using lubricants (such Into the Wylde) without glycerine, chlorhexidine, cyclomethicone, cyclopentasiloxane, cyclotetrasiloxane, mineral oil derivatives, nontoxynol 9, octoxynol 9, parabens, phthalates, polyquaternium 15, propylene glycol, sodium hydroxide, synthetic dyes or fragrances or triclosan, will help minimise irritation. Please also check the Therapeutics section later on for advice around menstrual wear. Surgery may be offered to remove some of the vestibular tissue, with the aim of removing some of the nerve endings. Sitz baths with nervines such as oat straw, as well as drinking nervine teas, may also help to normalise these over-stimulated nerves and pain receptors.

Suggested treatments: Therapeutics in the Nervines (p. 140) and Other lifestyle considerations (p. 169) sections would be specific here.

Cautions: Be aware that intimate pain can take a while to settle and it can be a disheartening process. Some of the journaling processes recommended further on in this book may be useful to accompany you through the process. It can also be reassuring to work with a therapist, whether psychosexual and/or a qualified professional complementary health practitioner to guide you through the process of re-wiring normal pain detection again. The nervines, mucosal membrane and anti-inflammatory categories of herbs in Part Four will be most useful for you here.

> Struggling with vulvodynia was a very lonely, hopeless experience. Eight years of going to doctors in three different countries and none of them could tell me what was happening. Then one day I was reading an article and the lady was describing symptoms I've been experiencing for all this time. Vulvodynia. I will never forget that feeling of knowing that I'm not the only one, and that I can be healed.

Then when I discovered I had vulvodynia I started researching ways to deal with it and I came across pelvic floor physiotherapy. I worked with a pelvic floor physio for the first 4–6 months and every week we had appointments, working to release trigger points with de-amouring, and retraining the brain–muscle–nerve connection. After a year after I was completely pain-free. All it took was some internal work, which was harrowing and heartbreaking, don't get me wrong. I also have pudendal neuralgia and hypertonic pelvic floor, so when I tense up now, I know what to do to relax the muscle and release the nerves in my pelvis.

It's a curable condition, but I know my case is different to someone else's. People might come to it from a background of repeated infections or unreleased trauma, for example. There is definitely stuff that can be done and it's not a lost cause. And you know what? That's amazing!!

—Oliwia

Vaginismus

What is it: Vaginismus is the over-tightening or contraction of the muscles of the vaginal wall, which can cause general discomfort, pain and difficulties during intercourse. Another name for it is levitator ani syndrome[10] and this refers to the Latin name for the collection of muscle groups involved. In fact, these muscles make up part of the pelvic floor and come together towards the back of the vestibule.

What symptoms are likely: Difficulty to achieve penetration in intercourse due to a tightness of the muscles, blocking access. It's also likely to cause some of the symptoms of provoked vestibulodynia as the tight muscles become tender. The blood flow in tight muscles is restricted and less oxygen is able to reach the muscle tissue. This results in a build-up of lactic acid in the muscle tissue (not in the vaginal mucous membrane!) and this causes the burning, rawness, throbbing, stabbing and aching, in a similar way to what happens when you get a stitch in an abdominal muscle after running.

What else it could be: It's worth testing for any of the other inflammatory, yet infectious conditions, as these can cause sensitisation and swelling in the area, which could imitate vaginismus.

More about it: Diagnosed by a physical examination, it is easily differentiated from any of the –dynia conditions mentioned above as it can be seen and felt by a diagnosing clinician. Electromyography and perineometry, which measure muscle tightness can also aid a diagnosis. Due to the tight nature of the pelvic floor muscles, women with vaginismus might also suffer from urinary urgency, increased frequency, incomplete emptying of the bladder, constipation haemorrhoids, rectal tears and lower back and hip pain.

How we get it: Lesions during delivery, reduced intra-vaginal discharge, menopause and psychological causes.

Approaches and aims: This is where a female health physiotherapist will come into their own, and whatever other therapeutics you try this should also form part of the picture. Aside from the physical therapy they provide, they may suggest biofeedback, heat therapy and dilators. The idea here is for your body to re-learn control and normal perception for the muscles involved. There are many types of dilators on the market and available from the NHS, and each person will have their own feelings on whether a particular set works well for them or not. I have heard that sets of vibrating dilators, starting from the slimmest size and working up are well tolerated and helpful in relearning appropriate responses to stimuli. These can be bought privately. Please see the Resources section.

Suggested treatments: Therapeutics in the Nervines (p. 140) and Other lifestyle considerations (p. 169) sections would be supportive here.

Vaginitis

Vaginitis is a term often used to describe non-specific pain and/or irritation in the vagina caused by inflammation. As we have seen above it can be caused by infection, but inflammation can also be caused without infectious agents present. Dermatitis can often be the cause in these cases and there are several types to consider:

Irritant contact dermatitis

This sort of dermatitis is very common and can account for up to 25% of vulvar irritation, burning and itching.[8] It is caused when the vulval tissues come into contact with a substance it finds irritating. This can be fabrics, soaps, menstrual products, toilet paper, laundry detergents.

Even cycling and rowing can cause this. Something to be mindful of is that any irritation and inflammation can make the tissues more prone to opportunistic infection.

Allergic contact dermatitis

Similar to the above, allergic contact dermatitis causes an immune system reaction, in which the irritated cells release histamine. This normally means that the symptoms can be worse than that of the 'irritant contact' type of dermatitis and can get worse upon each exposure to the offending material.

Chronic itching and scratching from any sort of vulvovaginal irritation can cause an immune reaction whereby mast cells release histamine in the area, leading to further irritation and a scratch/itch cycle that can take on a life of its own if it's not resolved. It can cause severe damage to the affected tissues, and women can often scratch in their sleep without realising the damage they are doing. This is called *Lichen simplex chronicus*.

With simple irritation it can be difficult to find the offending material and the best way to approach it is as you would an elimination diet, stripping everything back to basics. Wash with water (as you should be anyway!), use organic menstrual products, natural fabrics (organic if possible), and non-bio laundry liquid.

Keeping it simple for a period of time will allow your vulval tissue to recover and regain integrity, before any reintroduction. As you reintroduce something from your usual routine one at a time, it makes it easier to see what might be causing the irritation. Sometimes it can even be the toilet paper! More on that later. Just as this dermatitis can be present in the vagina, it can also be present on the vulva. If it appears in both, it is called vulvovaginitis.

Suggested treatments: In all cases of vaginitis or vulvovaginitis, a sitz bath with herbs from the Anti-inflammatory section (p. 119) would be a good approach. In cases of non-specific pain and/or irritation, a conventional/allopathic approach might be to prescribe a cream that contains Benzocaine. Benzocaine works by numbing the area, and we are told that it can burn on application, until the numbing action sets to work on your nerves. While this has the overall effect of stopping the pain and irritation for the time the cream is active (although it can cause irritation of its own accord) it doesn't address the reason the pain and irritation is present and does nothing to enrich the female experience. It is more a quietening or hushing of female pain rather than the satisfactory conclusion and discovery of the causative agents. To me this doesn't feel acceptable as a solution.

> I'm getting to a point when I own my vagina, rather than my vagina owning me.
>
> —Maddie

Vaginal prolapse

This is something to be aware of, particularly if you have given birth. Prolapse of a pelvic organ means that it slips down out of its normal position. Strain on the ligaments and musculature that keeps it in place can be the cause. Often it can be pelvic organs (uterus, bladder or bowel) that prolapse and bulge into the vagina. However, sometimes the vagina itself can prolapse, meaning that it becomes stretched, with reduced muscle tone to keep its normal shape. The downward collapse of the vaginal wall is called a vaginocele. It might present as a vulva that protrudes out with the labia minora stretched apart and the vaginal opening pulled apart (when normally they would appear closed).[16] In such a situation 'fanny farts', the unusual entry and expelling of air and water from swimming or bathing may make an ingress and egress, which may have an unfavourable effect on your vaginal microbiome.

Forming an awareness of your vaginal canal can be the first step in looking to treat this issue, and a trip to a female pelvic physiotherapist should definitely be on the cards. It's worth being informed about the options you may be offered conventionally. The vaginal mesh is now only offered in the UK on the NHS as a last resort, following the report of many devastating side effects of this treatment for pelvic organ prolapse and urinary incontinence, including pain, bleeding, bowel problems and difficulties with sexual intercourse.

Suggested treatments: Working with a pelvic health physio (cf. p. 179) can be vital here. Abdominal massage (cf. p. 114) can also be supportive. As with many of the conditions I mention, looking after the vaginal microbiome is key to boosting vaginal wellbeing so do check out the pH Modulation section (p. 153).

Inside out

A fullness, unaware.

Once held within.

Now newly conscious.

At the wonder of our feminine bodies.

Sadness.

At the changes, unexpected.

Joy at the reasons for it.

New paths, new body, new purpose.

Wisdom, compassion and love.

—Emny Kadri, Medical Herbalist

Fertility, pregnancy, miscarriage, birth and post birth

If you're thinking about trying to conceive or you are pregnant, it's worth thinking about your vaginal health, as certain aspects of it become more relevant. During pregnancy there is an increased blood flow to the area, meaning that the vulva can appear a darker colour. Progesterone rises, as does the glycogen content of the vaginal mucosal cells. These changes mean that the connective tissue in the area can relax and the muscles fibres in the wall of the vagina increase in size ready for birth.[17]

It can also mean that VVC (thrush) can be more prevalent in the second and third trimesters of pregnancy due to changes in the vaginal microbiome brought about through changed oestrogen and glycogen levels, as well as changes to the immune system.[18] Gestational diabetes may play a role here too, and it is worth monitoring blood sugar levels. If needed, pessaries to manage gestational VVC can be used up to two weeks before the due date and looking at ways to reduce the symptoms and ensure great blood sugar balance can be a way to approach it (cf. p. 173).

While a healthy maternal vaginal microbiome can be desirable in passing on good bacteria to a baby born by vaginal delivery, I think it's important to recognise the impact that the words 'good' or 'bad' can have on mothers, and rather concentrate on optimising the environment for the comfort of both mother and baby.

Research has shown links between the overgrowth of the anaerobic bacteria that causes BV, the aerobic bacteria that causes AV, Group *Strep B.* and *Mollicutes*, and an increased risk of infertility, pre-term birth, miscarriage and low birth weight. They are therefore often screened for.

Overall, having a healthy microbiome rich in *Lactobacilli* is one way to reduce all of these risks. Screening is often offered during pregnancy but, if you have any concerns, it's best to get these addressed before trying to conceive and certainly before your due date to improve overall outcomes.

During birth, the perineal and vaginal muscles relax and the vaginal rugae flatten to allow the vaginal canal to expand. Post birth it can take 6–12 weeks for the vagina to repair and return to its pre-birth dimensions, although this is just an estimate, so if it takes longer for you that's absolutely okay.

And so to discuss episiotomy and tearing. Episiotomy, now considered a 'standard' procedure is the deliberate cutting of the perineal tissue to avoid tearing of the area during birth. The idea being that cutting instead creates a more controlled wound to heal. While the process of birth allows the cervix and vagina to facilitate a baby, sometimes the baby comes quicker than the body has time to prepare for, or there are conditions that make tearing likely. Stitches are likely to be used.

It is also done if an instrumental birth is considered necessary. This would be when forceps or ventouse are used, and an episiotomy may be undertaken to get the instruments 'in'. These instruments are considered if there is a need to get the baby out quickly, often when it has been a long labour and the mother is tired. In many cases, using the force of gravity—which is impossible to do when lying on your back, but is how humans naturally give birth in a non-medicalised setting—would help to avoid the use of instruments.

If a Caesarean birth is planned or needed, there is growing evidence to suggest that 'seeding' the baby's face after delivery with a microbiome swab taken from the mother's vagina, as the baby would get via a vaginal birth, can help with the healthy development of the newborn's immune system.[19]

Approaches and aims: In preparation for birth there are some lovely natural massage balms out there specifically designed for perineal massage and this can help increase the flexibility and suppleness of this area. Healing following birth can be thought of in three different ways: tissue and muscular healing, nerve healing, and emotional processing and healing—these may overlap.

If tearing or episiotomy has occurred, a focus on healing the injured area involves keeping the area clean, and avoiding water until the body has started the repair work and it's no longer an open wound. During this time, it's important to avoid any activity that could traumatise the area, such as running or picking up something heavy. Sitting on an inflatable 'doughnut' to avoid pressure in the area is also a lovely idea.

Mother-roasting or -warming is a delightful sounding concept that was recommended historically for the 40 or so days 'sitting in' time until the bleeding after birth had finished. The mother is kept as warm as possible because warmth encourages blood flow, which in turn encourages healing. The traditional notion of keeping the feet warm to keep the uterus warm may also be part of this, as may pelvic wrapping, which has its origins in many traditional cultures around the world, but which is now attracting attention for potential cultural appropriation. However, it may be of benefit to the healing process.

Once the wound is starting to knit together well, use healing sitz baths of herbs such as *Calendula officinalis* for ten minutes daily, if you can, for up to six weeks, or simple Epsom salt baths with some lavender essential oil to improve healing and decrease scarring (see the Therapeutics section for more information on sitz baths). 'Padsicles', which are frozen maternity pads spritzed with witch hazel or aloe vera, and popped into your pants, can also be a massive comfort!

It's worth noting that although the general advice is to avoid intercourse for six weeks after a vaginal birth, and that tissue repair can take 6–12 weeks, it may take longer so don't worry if you're not fully healed by then. The way scar tissue forms means that the tissue feels tighter as the skin knits together. Due to this, your vagina and perineum may feel different and as far as intercourse is concerned you may need to mix things up a little bit to find positions and levels of penetration that work for the 'new' you, as you heal fully.

If things feel difficult and they are not improving, it might be very valuable to book in to see a women's pelvic health physio. These can be accessed privately or through the NHS and can be invaluable in aiding a full recovery after birth.

Emotional recovery is also important to be mindful of, especially as the transition period of becoming a new mum may leave little time to look after herself. Meditation and breathing exercises can be very helpful, but where ten minutes may feel unachievable and something to fail at, just two minutes fitted into a baby-led schedule can be beneficial. For processing any birth trauma, counselling, birth debriefing, 3-Step Rewind or EMDR can be helpful techniques that you can access professionally.

UTIs and the urinary tract microbiome

Urinary tract infections (UTIs) are very common (50% of all adult females and 10% of female children will have them at some point), and in adults it can have a causal relationship with sexual activity. Just as the digestive system and vagina have a microbiome, so, too, does the urinary tract. However, the urinary tract's microbiome has more similarity to the vaginal microbiome than it does to the digestive tract's. Often, the vaginal microbiome and the urinary tract microbiome can affect each other. It follows then that treating one can impact the other. The anatomical proximity of the urethra (where urine exits the body) and of the vagina is the rationale here, and they can share up to 60% of the same microbes in their microbiomes, with *Lactobacilli* dominating both in health.

The urinary tract also has a mycobiome that can include *Candida spp.* as well as other fungi such as *Aspergillus*, although in the vast majority of cases, bacterial infection with *E. coli* is to blame for acute UTIs. Symptoms of an acute lower UTI may include burning on urination, an increased frequency and urgency in passing urine. It's worth noting that some of these symptoms also can be experienced in menopause, with the absence of a UTI!

Chronic UTIs are a little more tricky to get to grips with as their symptoms can be harder to pin down, and on testing they often don't yield any positive results that would normally indicate infection. Symptoms may include bladder pain and kidney pain, and in these cases, diagnoses such as interstitial cystitis, overactive bladder syndrome and painful bladder syndrome are common (and trickier to deal with!).

Because of the overlap between the vaginal and the urinary tract microbiome, if chronic UTIs are becoming commonplace it's worth looking at what is going on with the vaginal health. Research in recent years has shown women with BV had higher rates of UTIs than those with a 'healthy' *Lactobacilli*-dominated vaginal microbiome,[20] and that some of the bacteria associated with BV can trigger dormant bacteria in the urinary tract to create a flare-up, disappearing without a trace while the infection is active.[21] These things are worth bearing in mind if UTIs are common for you!

Suggested treatments: Therapeutics in the Urinary (cf. p. 164) section would be specific here. The Antimicrobial section (p. 155) may offer supportive options here too.

Pelvic inflammatory disease (PID) and pelvic congestion syndrome (PCS)

PID is a serious condition that should not be left untreated as it can lead to infertility, abscess formation and toxic shock syndrome (TSS). It is an infection that can affect any part of the upper reproductive tract (cervix, uterus, fallopian tubes and ovaries) with the bacteria *Neisseria gohorrhoeae* and *chlamydiae* (which are responsible for STDs) as well as some of the bacteria involved in BV. Symptoms can include pain in the lower abdomen area, vaginal bleeding at irregular times, painful intercourse and may cause ectopic pregnancy. It's most common in women of reproductive age and can be confused with ectopic pregnancy. In severe cases, hospitalisation is required.

Pelvic congestion syndrome by contrast is chronic pelvic pain caused by enlarged or varicosed veins in the pelvic area and around the ovaries. The risk is higher for getting this if you have had children and diagnosis is by ultrasound, CT or MRI scan.

How to spot pelvic congestion

Very separate to PID and PCS, I wanted to mention a little about what pelvic congestion might mean when talking to a complementary health practitioner. In close proximity to the organs of the female reproductive tract we have the digestion tract, many blood and lymphatic vessels and lymph nodes (these are immune system hubs that look after and generate the immune cells in the blood). If digestion or the lymphatic drainage is sluggish, or anything affects the free flow of the blood in the blood vessels, the region may accumulate metabolic and environmental waste products. This would be termed 'pelvic congestion', and, in my clinical experience, can contribute to any recurrent or chronic vaginal condition. Assessment of this would be made in a consultation.

Suggested treatment: While PID and PCS require conventional intervention, supportive therapeutics alongside this include suggestions from the Digestion and elimination section (p. 132), the Immunity section (p. 124), and possibly abdominal massage (cf. p. 114).

STIs

STIs (sexually transmitted infections) are considered outside a herbalist's scope of practice to treat in the UK. That means that they absolutely have to be treated by a GP, and I need to impress the importance of this. A herbalist can, however, support someone who has an STI. This may come in the form of giving them herbal support for their immune and nervous systems, and restoration of their vaginal environment. However, this must be done in conjunction with conventional treatment from the GP.

Using condoms is really a point of self-care and should always be done, whether you are using another type of contraception or not, and even if you are in a long-term monogamous relationship. They massively reduce the risk of catching or passing on an STI, and will also help reduce the transmission of other microbes that affect vaginal health. Other people's intimate areas will have their own microbiomes, the composition of which will be different to yours, and they will affect yours when they come into contact. Sperm and seminal secretions have their own microbiome, as well as being more alkaline in pH, and these can affect your microbiome too. Open communication around using condoms before you get into a now or never situation can help set your boundaries clearly with the other party about what you are and aren't willing to do. At first, this might feel uncomfortable, but it is a great thing to do to care for yourself and your partner/s.

Another point of self-care is regular screening. Always do this between ending one relationship and starting another, and if you have multiple partners a more regular approach is advised. Test kits can now be ordered for free from the NHS (via https://sh24.org.uk) to do in the privacy of your home, so you don't necessarily need to go into a genitourinary medicine (GUM) clinic, and the results are texted to you.

With the explosion in the sex-tech scene there are some great apps out there that can help with screening (see Resources section for this, and for some great protection brands) and sharing your latest test results easily and confidentially with your partner/s, helping to break down the stigma around this area.

Below are the most common STIs with a brief description and symptoms. If you suspect you have any of these or think you might be at risk, please access screening services ASAP and if positive, go to your conventional healthcare provider in the first instance to seek treatment. You can always access complementary health routes to back up whatever conventional treatment you receive.

Gonorrhoea	A bacterial infection spread through sexual contact (not by kissing or hugging). You may have mild or no symptoms. Symptoms usually show up within a week of being infected and include pain on urination, yellow or bloody discharge and bleeding between your periods. It can be treated with antibiotics.
Syphilis	A bacterial infection spread by sexual contact that can cause permanent damage if not treated. It is very contagious. You may have mild or no symptoms. Symptoms may come and go over time, but this does not mean that the infection has been cleared. Symptoms come in stages that may overlap. Stage 1) a syphilis sore called a 'chancre' shows up where the infection entered your body. They are usually firm, round and painless and can also be open and wet. They can show up between three weeks to three months after you get the infection and can appear in hard to see places. They may also look like an ingrown hair or pimple. The chancre will last 3–6 weeks and will go away without treatment—however, *it still needs to be treated.*

(Continued)

	Stage 2) non-itchy rashes on the palm of your hands, soles of the feet or other areas will arise. The rashes sometimes can be hard to see. You may also feel nauseous and have flu-like symptoms. You can also have sores in your mouth, vagina and anus and have weight or hair loss. The rashes can last between 2–6 weeks and may come and go for up to two years.
	Stage 3) between stages two and three there may be long periods where you have no symptoms at all. The third stage is where serious health problems occur, including tumours, blindness and paralysis. This stage can still be treated, but the damage it has done to your body until this point cannot be changed or healed. It can be treated at any stage with antibiotics.
Chlamydia	A very common bacterial infection spread by sexual contact, and another one with often no or only mild symptoms, which can lead to infertility. Chlamydia can affect your eyes, if touched, or your throat. Symptoms include pain on urination, pain during intercourse, pain in your lower abdomen, a yellowish strong-smelling vaginal discharge, bleeding between periods, pain, discharge or bleeding around the anus.
HIV (Human Immunodeficiency Virus)	HIV is a virus that can lead to AIDS. It breaks down certain immune cells, meaning that you have a less robust response to infections which may lead to dying from a regular infection. Once you acquire HIV, you have it for life. AIDS is the disease that it can progress to, due to the damage HIV does to your immune cells. HIV can be passed by sexual contact. It can also be passed from

mothers to babies during pregnancy, birth or breastfeeding. Signs of AIDS include oral thrush, sore throat, vaginal thrush, PID, getting bad infections, tiredness, dizziness, light-headedness, headaches, weight loss, easy bruising, diarrhoea, fevers and night sweats, swollen glands in the throat, armpit or groin, deep dry coughing spells, shortness of breath, purplish areas on the skin or inside mouth, bleeding from the mouth, nose, anus or vagina, skin rashes, numbness of hands or feet and losing control of your muscles.

Pubic Lice (aka crabs)	Pubic lice are small parasites that attach to the skin and hair near your genitals. They are very common and passed on by prolonged contact. Symptoms appear about five days later and may include: a lot of itching in the genital area, tiny brown or whitish bugs in the pubic area (you may need a magnifying glass to see), oval, yellow or white eggs at the base of the pubic hair, dark or bluish areas where the lice are living, and feeling feverish, run down or irritable. Treatments come in topical gels, shampoos, liquids and foams.
Hepatitis B	Hep B is a liver infection caused by a virus that can be spread by sexual contact. It can be serious and there is no cure but can be prevented by using condoms. It is possible to have it without realising because in 50% of cases it has no symptoms. In the other 50%, symptoms can include feeling flu-like, fatigue, a pain in your stomach, losing your appetite, nausea and vomiting, pain in your joints, headache, fever, hives, dark-coloured urine, pale poo, yellowing skin and whites of eyes.

(*Continued*)

Herpes	Herpes is a viral infection that stays with you for life. It causes oral and genital sores, which can be painful but don't usually lead to serious health problems. There is no cure, but there is medication that can ease symptoms and lower your chances of passing the virus onto others. There will be periods when you don't have any symptoms, but you will still have the virus and it can still be passed on. The sores it causes come as a group of itchy or painful blisters on the vaginal, vulva, cervix, anus or inside of the thighs. Other symptoms may include a burning sensation if your urine touches a herpes sore, difficulty in urination if a blister is blocking your urethra and flu-like symptoms. The first outbreak is usually the worst and can last from 2–4 weeks. Subsequent break-outs can be shorter and fewer.
Trichomoniasis	Trichomoniasis or 'trich' for short, is caused by a parasite that is carried in semen and vaginal discharge. It's the most common curable STI and is treated by antibiotics. Seventy per cent of people won't show symptoms, but when symptoms do appear one of the most common is vaginitis (inflammation of the vagina) with a green/grey/yellow, frothy and or bad-smelling discharge, and it can cause pain on and increased frequency and urgency of urination. Other symptoms include blood in the vaginal discharge, itching and irritation around the vagina, pain on intercourse and swelling around the genitals. Symptoms can range from mild to painful and can start from three days to a month after exposure. Note that symptoms can be so similar to AV or a UTI that testing is important to determine what is going on.

Molluscum contagiosum	A viral infection that causes small bumps on the skin. Contracted by touching infected skin or sharing things like towels or clothing and isn't confined to sexual contact; often children can have it too as we have seen above (on non-genital areas) and it is very contagious. Characterised by small firm bumps on the skin that have a dimple in the middle. They are usually flesh-coloured. They are often treated in a similar way to warts and left untreated they can take 6–12 months to clear up on their own.

While this is just a whistle-stop tour of STIs, I appreciate that it's quite a scary one. Growing up in the 1980s, the public information films the government put out to educate everyone about AIDS really informed and tainted my view of sex, and I can wholly appreciate the information presented here could also have the same effect, to a lesser extent. However, it is important to cover STIs so as to understand this set of conditions. With the correct risk management (screening) and control measures (condoms anyone?!) you can keep yourself and your partner/s safe. See the Resources section for some suggestions for condoms, screening and dental dam brands.

A word about antibiotics

As this is a book about natural approaches you may have been surprised to see antibiotics mentioned here—so a small word about them. While antibiotics can trigger episodes of VVC and upset the microbiome balance (because antibiotics kill microbes, often indiscriminately), in some cases, such as STIs, it can prove to be lifesaving medicine. Therefore, antibiotics aren't discriminately bad. Sometimes they are necessary and needed, and if they are, we can then address the imbalances they cause and repair any damage to the microbiome following their use.

You may have also heard about antibiotic resistance. This is when a class of antibiotics becomes less able to kill a microbe across a population due to their overuse for minor issues, or their misuse when other treatments might be just as effective. Their overuse causes the microbes to become resistant to them, meaning that we are in danger of losing the usefulness of this class of lifesaving medicines. To help combat this, only use antibiotics if really necessary. It's a good idea to find out what else could be used in milder situations where a GP may routinely hand out antibiotics (such as colds). Talk to your professional registered complementary healthcare provider for some guidance.

What to do when symptoms or results are unclear and things just feel a little off

In many cases, symptoms might not fit into a clear picture of what's going on. Maybe you can relate to some of the symptoms identified above, but not all for a condition, or you have a mix of symptoms, or you have very slight symptoms which are affecting your comfort either daily or at certain points in your cycle.

Be assured that this is very normal. The presentations of conditions that affect vaginal health can be very confusing, and it may be outside your scope of expertise using information from this book to work out exactly what is going on.

It is true that certain vaginal conditions can exist concurrently, that is, together, and/or that they can occur in swift succession straight after each other, thus muddying the picture and confusing you. It's often worth thinking about getting a swab test done and an STI screening just to rule things out. It's also worth considering whether you have any other allergies as this can often translate into a vaginal effect too (think mucous membranes), whether you own any animals (which may cause allergies), and whether you have any other systemic conditions such as Diabetes or Behçet's syndrome, as these could all play a role.

If you feel unclear about what is going on for you, do go to the GP and get a swab test in the first instance. A home pH test might also come in handy (this and the swab results certainly will be if you book into see me!) to give a generalised idea of the environmental conditions that are going on there.

How a health system reports on the results of a vaginal swab varies from country to country, and in the UK this can even vary from primary care trust to primary care trust. However, they are a good starting point in the detective work that is needed for tricky situations. I say starting point, because if you get inconclusive results, results that don't show the presence of any pathogen, or your body isn't 'responding' to standard treatment as your GP might expect, it just means that we haven't yet got to the root cause of what is going on. Don't take these kind of results as a last chance saloon for getting answers—there is more we can do, and it may involve going to see a qualified registered complementary health practitioner that specialises in vaginal health!

> I
> think that
> SHAME HARMS
> vaginas in so many
> different ways & forms
> it erodes our own self as well
> Society told me I was 'less than' for
> having one   that I was
> without. That   vaginal
> pleasure is   wrong.
> That vaginas   are
> sinful, smelly   unclean.
> This is shame   but it is
> shame that is   wrong. It
> is shame that   must be put
> right. When I   had swelling
> pain and UTI   symptoms for
> months and Dr's   kept giving me
> antibiotics. It was   bubbles
> in my bath.   Soap as well.
> I had subscribed   to the idea
> that I needed to   be clean
> down there.   I didn't.
> the vagina   is self
> cleaning.   Which is
> pretty amazing. It
> was this that woke
> me up to harm
> and also to
> shame.

—Kelly Johnson

In fact, sometimes when you have a discharge that's unusual to you, but your culture and microscopy swabs come back without a definitive cause, nothing abnormal is showing or you are told that it is normal physiology or all in your head, these new tools can come in handy!

One of the new tools that has come out in the last few years is the microbiome testing kit. Usually developed, sold and processed by testing laboratories used by practitioners, they utilise the latest in PCR and DNA profiling of all the organisms in someone's vaginal microbiome to analyse and identify exactly what's there. This is all done by analysis of what is actually found to be present rather than requiring culturing (growing in the lab) and microscopy (counting what has grown under the microscope). Some tests can even measure the level of inflammation present.

A word of advice on these though: if you are keen to get one of these done, remember that it is just a snap-shot in time of what is going on in your vaginal microbiome. The microbiome is a dynamic environment that is changing all the time, and does not stay static—so do it when your symptoms are at their worst! And do them through a practitioner that is trained to analyse the results, because it can be very confusing to do this yourself and is really not advisable. The tests aren't cheap but are worth it if it's unclear what is going on for you and need to be read by someone who understands what they are saying.

The neo-vagina and likely conditions

Although there isn't as much data known yet for people with neo-vaginas (although this is growing all the time), the conditions most likely to cause issues are prolapse, a short vaginal canal, difficulty in passing urine, and vaginal discharge.[22] Due to the nature of much of the original tissue (scrotal) that is used to create the neo-vagina and associated structures, hair growth can cause a problem, even after the recommended electrolysis. It may disrupt the bacterial composition of the area and cause a foul-smelling discharge. In this case, further electrolysis is often recommended along with douching (something that is not recommended for natal vaginas!!!) to help keep the area bacterially healthy.

Regular use of dilators is recommended to avoid prolapses, and to maintain girth and depth of the neo-vagina. In some cases, further surgery may be offered to attempt to improve any narrowing or shortening here.[22] It has also been reported that there may be an increased risk of squamous cell carcinoma[9] associated with the creation of neo-vaginas, and although that is outside the scope of this book, it's something worth bearing in mind.

Suggested treatments: Overall supporting the body with Therapeutics in the Immunity (p. 124) and Nervines (p. 140) sections would be helpful here, alongside conventional treatment.

How intercourse impacts vaginal health

This section explores what happens to and with the vagina during intercourse. Of course, not all sex involves penetrative intercourse, and not all intercourse involves penis-in-vagina, but this section is more or less about penis-in-vagina intercourse as this can cause the most dramatic effect on the vaginal environment.

As we know, the vaginal pH is on the acidic end of the pH scale, nominally sitting at around 4–4.5 (although there can be variances in this that can be happily tolerated and considered normal). The pH of seminal fluid and sperm is a little more alkaline at around pH6. If these two have contact (either in unprotected sex, or in trying to conceive) the penile and seminal microbiome and pH can have an impact on the vaginal microbiome, as it stays in the area for some time. The more alkaline pH of the sperm may alter the vaginal pH and make it more susceptible to BV-causing microbes (have you ever noticed a slightly fishy smell after vaginal sex?—it'll be due to that—again, it's not a cleanliness issue). So it's worth taking this into account.

Obviously, not all intercourse involves penis-in-vagina. However, the microbiome of all the partners involved interact and have an impact on each other, and this includes the use of sex toys. This is something to think about when undertaking sex with a new partner—you will share your microbial colonies with your partner and vice versa, whatever genitalia are involved. Bear this in mind if any changes occur with your intimate health around this time. If this does adversely impact on you, panic not—it is possible to look at influencing both your and your partner's intimate microbiomes to improve the situation.

The sexual response, arousal, and libido

Libido, arousal and response are an area where body and brain come together (pun absolutely intended) in concert to orchestrate the sexual response, and this, of course, affects the sexual organs, including the vagina.

As humans we might have expectations, both of our own and that of society, around what our libido and readiness for sexual activity should look and feel like. However, as I think we have seen by now, I am a real advocate for breaking down those 'shoulds' and instead leaning into what our body, mind, feelings and emotions are actually telling us, within legal and ethical frameworks—for those things can never be wrong and can rather act as our guide for how we present and act in the world.

Libido is defined as sexual desire or sex drive. This doesn't need to be in relation to another person and is actually just your own level of desire to be engaged in a sexual activity (whether solo or partnered). Many factors can feed into or modify your libido, including hormone levels, where you are in your menstrual cycle if pre-menopausal (testosterone is the hormone classically considered the main one in determining sex drive—and yes, women have this hormone too, but ratios of oestrogen and progesterone also play a role), stress levels and other factors including medication, cortisol levels, being distracted with other things, mood and serotonin levels, and age or life stage. Your sex drive is really how your brain and body come together to determine your interest in sex at any given time.

The sexual response is a very physical one. Arousal is the body's response to mental, emotional and physical stimuli and causes increased heart rate, blood pressure and rate of breathing or respiration, as well as the dilation of blood vessels through the release of nitric oxide, which plays a role in erectile tissue infusion and vaginal lubrication. This stimulus is individual to each of us and the process enables the tissues of these organs to engorge with blood, heightening sensitivity and ability to feel pleasure, which produces a positive feedback loop. These tissue sites include the nipples, clitoris, labia and vagina. The vagina is then lubricated, mainly by fluid produced and excreted by the Batholin's glands, and to a lesser extent the Skene's glands, to join any mucous already present.

This stimulus also brings about changes in brain chemistry via various sets of neurotransmitters, or as I prefer to think of them, molecules of bliss, lighting up various pleasure-centres in the brain at different points in the process. In the initial stages of arousal, dopamine is queen, boosting your experience of pleasure and motivating you to seek out pleasurable and rewarding activities.

The second 'textbook' stage of arousal, also known as the plateau phase, takes place from the initiation of sexual contact until orgasm. In this stage the tissues swell even more, the clitoris becomes more sensitive, the muscles in the vagina tighten and the opening of the vagina becomes more narrow. This is a textbook description—you may find your experience differs from this, and that is absolutely fine.

During orgasm, vaginal lubrication increases, with increased activity from your Skene's glands. The muscles in your vaginal walls, and possibly in other areas in your pelvic floor or body, contract and release in pleasurable waves. A variety of neurotransmitters are released at orgasm, which contribute to that pleasure.

– **Oxytocin:** released by the hypothalamus and known as the love or cuddle hormone, oxytocin plays a role in bonding between two people, either through sex, or between a mother to baby (it is also involved in uterine contractions in labour and is stimulated during breastfeeding for the same reason, helping to return the uterus to its normal, pre-pregnancy size). In men, oxytocin may play a role in sperm movement and testosterone production. And in women, oxytocin continues to be released after orgasm, which may explain the wish for post-coital cuddles.
– **Prolactin:** this hormone peaks after orgasm, and in women is normally associated with breastfeeding, but in sex, studies show it seems to have a correlation with sexual satiety.
– **Endorphins:** our natural pain-killing hormones, endorphin surges normally accompany the release of oxytocin, thereby making you much less sensitive to pain during sex. A strange but interesting fact is that orgasm and pain may activate some of the same areas in the brain!
– **Serotonin:** another hormone, serotonin is released by the brain after orgasm and is known to have antidepressant qualities, promoting good mood, relaxation and peacefulness. It may also be the reason you feel sleepy after orgasm. Following any orgasm the body relaxes again.

Now, this isn't a researched piece of evidence and I can't back it up, but I wonder—the conventional notion is that men have a higher sex drive or libido than women, but when I talk to the women I know both personally and professionally, this doesn't stack up. In many cases women are exhibiting a higher sex drive than their male partners, and this is often flagged by who is initiating sexual contact. This might be for any number of reasons (perhaps the male partners might not want to feel as though they are 'harassing' their female partners for sex), but I think it's time to well and truly discard the myth that men's sex drives are higher than women's. An interesting topic for research if anyone wants to pick that up...

A place for aphrodisiacs

It's such a seductive idea to use herbs as aphrodisiacs and is in fact one of the most famed ways that they have been employed over the centuries. How does the idea of experimenting with aphrodisiacs feel to you?

It can be a fun way to enhance and play with your libido and in some cases can help revitalise a repressed or 'asleep' sense of sexual desire (although there are other aspects to look at too—they are not there to force or cajole the body to respond how you want it to—as we've seen in the section above, there are so many aspects and inputs to your sexual response).

What ways could a herb act as an aphrodisiac? Well, it could be through increasing your vital energy so that your body has enough resources to invest in sex and reproduction (which is after all its biological function); it could be through helping your body to manage stress levels; it could be through modulating your sex hormones; it could be through exciting the senses, such as smell, sight and touch, allowing you to connect more deeply with your sensuality.

It's important to note that aphrodisiacs shouldn't be used without any participants' consent or if you aren't really into the idea of it. It's not that they act against the body and force it to have responses that aren't welcome—as, with hypnotherapy, it works with your will, not in spite of it. I see them as a 'fun' addition to the menu. Their energies can be subtle or more obvious. In the Therapeutics section (p. 140) you will find some suggestions for aphrodisiacs. Have fun (if you'd like to).

Orgasm

Several physiological aspects are involved in orgasm in the female-anatomised body, and orgasm can be triggered or stimulated by involvement of one or a number of these areas. If more than one area is involved, it is known as a blended orgasm.

- **The clitoral orgasm:** this is probably the most common body part stimulated in the female orgasm, and the type of orgasm that Freud in his infinite wisdom (don't get me started) termed as an immature orgasm. Clitoral orgasm can be triggered by the stimulation of the exposed head of the clitoris, known as the glans clitoris (as referred to in the earlier chapter), which is often the 'go-to' for the self-pleasured orgasm. However, as we've seen from looking at the anatomy earlier, the bulb of vestibule and crus both wrap around the vaginal canal and so internal stimulation of these parts of the clitoris may be involved in penetrative stimulation.

- **G spot:** the G spot (also known as the Goddess Spot in some circles, although the G stands for Gräfenberg, after yet another male doctor) is thought to be an internal part of the clitoris or urethral sponge that lies close to the anterior (front) vaginal wall. There has even been some debate historically as to whether the G spot exists (please bear in mind that until the late 1980s the full anatomy of the clitoris wasn't mapped or even understood—insert eye roll here). To locate yours, insert a clean finger or two into your vagina and curl forwards to the front of the vaginal wall. There is an area of rougher or bumpier feeling tissue—this is your G spot. Stimulation of this spot causes the tissue to become engorged with blood. It has been reported to produce impressive-feeling orgasms as well as an empirical association with the phenomenon of 'squirting' (ejaculating fluid produced by the Skene's glands from the urethra due to orgasm). Anyone who has had a G spot stimulated orgasm knows this area is no myth!

- **AFE spot:** similar to the G spot, the anterior fornix erogenous spot, resides again on the anterior (front) vaginal wall, a lot higher/deeper and closer to the cervix than the G spot. Made of the same erectile tissue as the G spot, and possibly attributed to the urethral sponge, when stimulated it can help produce lubrication and contribute to orgasm. There may be other erogenous areas deep within the vaginal canal which haven't yet been verified by research. However, if something feels right, we can't deny its existence.

- **Cervical orgasm:** kind of does what it says on the tin but can be elusive because the cervix can hold what can best be described as tension due to emotional disturbance such as trauma (both physical or mental/emotional), causing numbness or pain on contact. With care, this can be reduced through a process called de-armouring (a little more on this in the paragraph below) until the feeling of pleasure can be detected on loving and respectful contact with this miraculous site in our bodies.

Toys can be used to find and stimulate these deeper orgasm zones within the body and help you work out what you like in self-play, which can then help you communicate to your partner what works for you in partnered play. There are several shaped glass, body-safe ceramic or crystal dildos that can be great for this type of exploration. They may also be used in cervical mapping and de-armouring work—best done with the guidance of a qualified practitioner experienced in this practice. Check the Resources section for suggestions.

A note on cervical health, smears, HPV, dysplasia, pleasure and de-armouring

I thought long and hard about whether to include the cervix in this book. Considered to be anatomically separate from the vagina (it is, after all, part of the uterus, and rests atop of the vaginal canal), it even has its own microbiome! However, it shares part of the same space as the vaginal canal and does in fact, terminate the end of the vaginal space. The cervix responds to hormonal fluctuations and gently rises up and down within the vaginal cavity depending on where you are in your cycle, if indeed cycling.

I want to cover it briefly here. However, there is enough information known and written about the cervix to fill an entire book in its own right—and this is what some people have done (recommended further reading in the resource list).

As the doorway and gatekeeper to and from the uterus, the health and pleasure of the cervix, metaphorically—both spiritually and physically—can be thought of to do with permission and what we allow into and out of our intimate space. It allows sperm in; and menstrual blood, pregnancies that did not make it to full term, and babies to come out. It is literally a gateway of human life, a threshold and a boundary. Bear with me on this and allow yourself to go with the analogy for a while, do a little further reading around it, and, of course, do come up with your take on this.

In the UK, the NHS has a cervical screening programme that routinely allows for a smear or pap test for everyone with a cervix between the ages of 25 and 64. Nominally, it happens every three years up until the age of 50 and then it moves to every five years. As part of the test, a speculum is inserted into the vagina and opened so that the clinician can find your cervix. A small stiff brush-like instrument is used to collect a small sample of cells from around the cervical os (opening).

If an abnormal result is found (abnormal meaning the test reveals cell changes), further investigations are made, which may result in increased frequency of testing, a colposcopy (a visual inspection of the face of the cervix, performed in a hospital), or a variety of treatments designed to remove abnormal cells, until a normal result is recorded.

It is through these screenings that HPV, dysplasia (pre-cancerous cell changes) and cancerous cell changes are found and graded so that monitoring and treatment can be administered. HPV is a family of viruses that are sexually transmitted but can lie dormant for years before expressing themselves. Fourteen of the virus variants have been linked to developing cervical cancer, and this is why it is now routinely tested for in the UK.

I want to be clear that it's my opinion that cervical screening is absolutely essential and saves lives (for those of us old enough to remember Jade Goody in the UK). However, I also recognise that these screenings aren't popular, comfortable, dignified or in any way pleasant. They may also provide understandable additional challenges for people who have been sexually abused, assaulted or identify as trans or non-binary.

While acknowledging the importance of the testing, and advocating for those who find the test a particular challenge, it must be noted that the physical way the test is set up (patient on a couch, spot light on our intimate areas and legs splayed wide) is very much set up for the convenience of the medical professional rather than for the convenience and comfort of the patient. The emphasis is on the ease of obtaining the sample, and it can be disempowering for the person being tested. While having the test and knowing your results is very much an empowered choice that puts your health firmly in your hands, front and centre, the way it is set up makes us feel, as the patient, out of control and secondary to the process. We are not. It is for our health, and with this in mind I want to stand with you side by side in voicing any concerns to your healthcare professional as they perform the test.

Perhaps the angle they are inserting the speculum at is uncomfortable, or it would be more bearable for you if they used a smaller size speculum, or slowed down. During sexual penetration, it is not comfortable for us if our bodies are not ready, and the concept of permission and care should be central to this type of testing. Do not feel bad for asking your clinician to work in a way that makes it better for you. Maybe you would like to see your cervix—you could even ask if it would be possible to do this while the clinician has the speculum inserted and the cervix located. Bring a handheld mirror to have a look!

As we have seen above, the cervix can also be a source of pleasure through orgasm, but may also hold and somatise trauma through 'armouring', which I read as 'protecting' the cervix from feeling more trauma which may prevent that pleasure from being felt. It may present as pain and numbness. There are practitioners who can assist you in 'mapping' and 'de-armouring' your cervix, allowing stored trauma to be released from the area, allowing for a full expression of pleasure from this wonderful part of female-bodied anatomy. Please see the Resources section to find out more.

Considerations

When thinking about sexual interactions and menstrual health, here are some areas you may want to take into consideration when choosing what's best for you.

Sexual health status and testing: in the UK, the standard NHS tests delivered via the SH:24 service are for *Chlamydia*, *Gonorrhoea* and *Syphilis*—and you can request an HIV test too. The tests are ordered discretely online and delivered to your home where DIY test samples can be collected (urine sample for men and swab for women, as well as a blood test) and sent back. These services are great as they rule out some of the more severe and even life-threatening conditions. However, they do not test for all STIs and can't account for many of the microbes that can play havoc with your vaginal health, so using a condom for any penile/penetrative sex is still advised to minimise disturbance to your vaginal ecology.

It's also important to break down the language around your sexual health status. Testing negative for STIs is traditionally associated with the words 'clean' or 'clear' and I think this adds to the negative stigma around sex in general. The sexual health testing service iPlaySafe have done some wonderful work around the stigma of these words, which is well worth checking out.

Lubricants: being the founder of the lube company Into the Wylde, I have a lot to say about this. Lubricants can mean *everything* when it comes to having a comfortable penetrative experience as a woman, meno-pausal or not! Where to start? First, I want to break down the myth that only menopausal or post-menopausal women need to use lubricant in sex. Need is a divisive word and I feel here we miss some of the nuance that lubricant can provide. There are many reasons besides menopause that women could benefit from increased or enhanced lubrication for penetrative sex. Vaginal and vulval tissue can be damaged with micro-traumas and abrasions if the area isn't lubricated to an ideal level when penetration occurs.

There are many reasons our bodies may not have provided optimal levels of lubrication by the time penetration occurs, and there is absolutely nothing wrong with you if you haven't. Your body is not broken or defective. It's normal. Reasons for this might include: penetration happening before enough foreplay has occurred to allow optimal lubrication to happen; hormone level fluctuations including post-natally and at certain points in your cycle which are naturally 'dryer'; being sub-optimally hydrated; heaters on in the room you are in; medication, including for hay fever (designed to dry up mucosal membranes) and for depression and anxiety (which modify some of the neurotransmitters that are concurrently involved in arousal and orgasm); scarring or trauma to the area involved, including from medical procedures or giving birth; you have a cold or minor infection; you are pregnant; you are on hormonal medication; or you are using a soap or perfume which can cause dryness (see the next section).

Now you understand why there's nothing wrong with you after all, and that many factors may be affecting how lubricated you are. It's totally normal to experience dryness from time to time, and using a good lubricant enhances and prolongs pleasure (doesn't just fix a problem). It may make it easier to orgasm, help sex to last longer, decrease pain and reduce micro tears and abrasions in the vaginal tissues—thereby reducing the number of opportunistic infections by organisms such as *Candida* spp. and *Gardnerella* (also STIs).

Adding lubrication is a very simple and effective way to immediately enhance penetrative sex, but it's got to be a good quality lube with good quality ingredients and properties, that are suitable for your needs. This brings me nicely onto my next point: what to look for in a lube. Anywhere between 60–80% of the chemicals from products that you put onto your skin, and indeed go in your vagina, are absorbed by the bloodstream.

As we have already seen, the vagina has a very specific ecology that is designed to keep the area healthy and trouble-free, and this is where the ingredients of your lube product really matter. Ingredients like glycerine are well documented as providing a food source for any opportunistic fungal microbes that are more than likely hanging out in your vagina. Here's a list of a few ingredients that can be found in some of the big commercial lubes that you might want to think twice about using.

Chlorhexidine	An antibacterial agent, which can indiscriminately disrupt healthy vaginal flora.
Glycerine	Found in most intimate lubricants—feeds the fungus *Candida albicans*, even at low concentrations. *Candida albicans* is responsible for most cases of vaginal thrush. Glycerine also increases the osmolarity of a lube, making damage to vaginal mucosa more likely, and therefore more susceptible to opportunistic infection by *Candida* spp. or *Gardnerella vaginalis*.
Mineral Oils and derivatives	Oils derived from crude oil production. These are used in the traditional cosmetic industry due to their skin-like feel and economic price. However, they can break down condoms and cause intimate irritation, increased risk of infection and changes in vaginal pH.
Nonoxynol 9	A detergent and surfactant (often included in cosmetics for its emulsifying properties) which was found to 'punch' holes in the cell membrane of sperm, thereby making it suitable for use as a spermicide. However, it is so good at breaking down cell membranes that it may also have the same effect on vaginal cell membranes, increasing risk of infection.
Octoxynol 9	A detergent and surfactant which may cause irritation and endocrine disruption.
Parabens	A family of synthetic preservatives found in many cosmetics and personal care products which may have a link to hormone disruption.
Phthalates	Plasticisers found in a whole host of cosmetics and plastic toys. Some of these are suspected endocrine/hormone disrupters and may be linked to reproductive toxicity and fertility issues.
Polyquaternium 15	Sometimes found in water-based lubricants, this positively-charged polymer, appeared to actively increase HIV replication in cell cultures in one study, and therefore could raise one's risk of HIV transmission.

Propylene Glycol	This is a synthetic liquid substance that absorbs water and is also used as an anti-freeze in the food, chemical and pharmaceutical industries. May cause allergic contact dermatitis, with a higher incidence in those with eczema or fungal infections.
Sodium Hydroxide	Also known as lye and caustic soda, this is a strongly alkaline substance.
Synthetic Dyes	Substances that confer colour. They may cause irritation on exposure to intimate mucosal membranes and skin.
Synthetic Fragrances	Substances that confer scent. Often a combination of products of unknown toxicity and allergy, they often cause vaginal irritation and therefore higher susceptibility to infection.
Triclosan	An antibacterial preservative, which may be associated with hormone disruption.

As we know pH is also an issue, so look for a lubricant that has a pH of around 4, to match your intimate happy pH levels. You might also want to consider whether having an organic or vegan product also fits with your desires.

Here are some further aspects to think about when choosing a lube:

Do you use barrier-method contraception such as condoms?
In this case you should be using a water or silicon-based lube.

Are you using a toy?
Then make sure you use a water-based lube, as silicone-based lubes could degrade the surface of a toy, especially if it's made from silicone—if in doubt, go for water-based.

Are you trying to conceive?
Then make sure you use a lube that is pro-conception—the pH of sperm is much higher (at around pH6) and a pro-conception lube will have matching pH. It is worth bearing in mind that these lubes may irritate your vagina because of these pH issues, but you may want to use these nevertheless.

Are you going to go anal?
A silicone or thick, water-based lube may be better here. Silicone lasts longer than a water-based one, and oil wouldn't be suitable here due to

the use of condoms (a barrier method that helps prevent the transmission of any potential HIV).

Different types of lube:

Water
Good for use in virtually all situations, water-based lubricants are safe for use even with condoms and toys and generally won't stain your sheets.

Oil
Very long-lasting, has a low re-application rate, and is useful for massage too—just not for condom use! It can also play havoc with vaginal pH.

Silicone
Long-lasting and often hypo-allergenic, this is suitable when having sex in water and anal sex. Definitely not suitable for use with toys!

Hybrid
These lubes are water-based with a small amount of silicone, making a creamy texture, which combines the best aspects of both types, with long-lasting lubrication and versatility. Some may be suitable for use with toys but always do a patch test first!!! As all sex is generally better with (the right) lube, it's a good idea to find one that you're happy with that doesn't cause you any problems and you can use liberally, with love.

Condoms: minimise the risk of sharing intimate infections and microbes; protects against STIs and prevents the passing backwards and forward of vaginal thrush or BV if you are trying to clear it up. There are condoms made from different materials on the market so if one type doesn't agree with you or your partner's intimate areas, there are many more to try.

Toys: a wonderful addition to self-pleasure or partnered activities. Make sure to always carefully wash toys after use; not share toys; use ones made from body-safe materials; match the correct sort of lube for the toy, i.e. not a silicone lube if the toy is made from silicone as it can dissolve the material the toy is made from; and use a thicker lube if the toy is intended for anal play.

Hygiene matters: this is a big topic and one that I don't think is spoken about or is clear enough in our society. This stuff isn't routinely taught to us growing up—and I think it should be. The vagina has been designed to be, on the whole, self-cleaning. This means that soap isn't needed on the vulva or in the vagina when you wash. In fact, it's best not to use it. It can seem like soaps and intimate washes might have a place in our bathrooms, after all, they seem like basic hygiene items. But no. Although some are specifically marketed for intimate hygiene, all soaps, especially fragranced ones, will knock our intimate pH and vaginal microbiome out of balance, which can cause mild itching, thrush and bacterial vaginosis.

Instead, use soap or shower gel on the mons or outside parts that have hair—all the labia needs is washing with plain water. The vagina never needs washing—it cleans itself! As a rule of thumb, the areas that have naturally got hair you can wash with a gentle soap or gel. Anything inside or beyond that only need a rinse with warm water as you are washing, and never use water in the vagina. That includes douching. Just don't. Whatever has happened, your body doesn't need it and it will only disrupt your natural microbial balance.

Even if you have a touch of vaginal thrush or BV and you want to just feel 'clean' there and wash away the discharge—please only wash the vulva with water. You can use a clean cloth or flannel if you feel that would help (making sure it's only been washed in non-bio laundry detergent). Please ignore all the intimate washes that are advertised to us, especially for sensitive or itchy times, or heaven forbid to make us smell 'nice'—they are likely to make matters worse.

When wiping after using the toilet, wipe front to back to avoid cross-contamination from the anus to the urethral/vaginal area and vice versa. While we are talking about hygiene, I want to talk about smell. Your intimate area is meant to have a smell. That smell can change over the month and is naturally light and musky. This is not something to feel embarrassed about—we're meant to smell this way and it can be a turn-on for an intimate partner. Once you accept and make friends with your natural smell, you can use it to help detect if something isn't right, such as tending towards a 'fishy' smell if you have BV or 'yeasty/ bready' if you have a fungal infection.

Peeing after sex: this brings us nicely onto peeing after sex. Doing this as soon as is realistic following intercourse can help avoid UTIs if you are prone to them. It may help to 'flush out' any unfriendly microbes that may have made their way into the urethral area during sexual activity before they have a chance to cause an issue. This isn't a clinical imperative. This is just a suggestion. Try it and see if it makes a difference for you.

Smoking: smoking is a risk factor. That is, it has been shown to likely increase the incidence of bacterial vaginosis. It has an anti-oestrogenic effect in the body, which may affect the health and prevalence of the beneficial *Lactobacilli* bacteria. Trace amounts of benzo[a]pyrene-diol-epoxide (BPDE) have been found in the vaginal secretions of smokers, and may affect the health of the *Lactobacillus*. Ostensibly, smoking increases the risk of vaginal dysbiosis.[23]

Obesity: research indicates that there might be a correlation between obesity and vaginal dysbiosis.

Immune health: the immune system is a complex collection of physical tissue barriers, organs and cells designed to protect the body from foreign pathological substances. When our immune system is working optimally it fights infection, which includes vaginal infection. There has been research[65] which shows that certain components of the immune system involved in the inflammatory process can be implicated in recurrent thrush, for example, and clinically I have seen a correlation between helping a client to improve their immune health and a resolution or reduction in frequency of these recurrent types of vaginal conditions. There are a variety of elements that can affect the effectiveness of our immune health, including: environmental, chemical or emotional stress—which can down-regulate certain elements of the immune system; quality of diet (is our diet providing enough of the building blocks we need to keep us healthy such as vitamins C and D); co-infection (which adds further work for the immune system to do when already under stress); thyroid health; genetics; autoimmunity (which is a form of immune dysregulation, when the immune system stops recognising the body as 'self' and starts targeting specific aspects of it as though it is a foreign pathological substance); and steroid use.

A quick way to assess your immune system is to see how many common colds you get during the year, and how your body responds. Few colds coupled with a robust (strong) response and swift resolution would be a fair indication that your immune system is broadly functioning well. Something less than this and you may wish to use some of the therapeutics in Part Four to improve your outcomes.

Menstrual protection: with many options of menstrual protection now available and widely used (such as disposable pads and tampons, organic options, washable and reusable pads, menstrual cups and discs, and period underwear), I really only give advice around this when there seems to be a hypersensitivity issue behind any recurrent vaginal health issues people are having. If using disposables, organic is always better—did you know there is no law to state that the chemical ingredients found in menstrual wear needs to be listed, and various studies have found them to contain multiple chemicals, such as dioxins, that I would not be happy to have next to my most intimate parts. However, if hypersensitivity is coming up then I would suggest switching to a menstrual cup, if you like using something insertable, or reusable pads or pants if you favour pads, as less or no fibres will be present to irritate your mucosa. Some may even choose to free bleed, while for others blood needs to be 'caught' higher up to stop it aggravating a sensitivity issue.

While there is no one product that is universally well tolerated by everyone, one thing to bear in mind with reusables and washables is that it is a good idea to change them every few months to reduce any potential bacterial load that could knock your intimate ecology out. When choosing a new type of menstrual product it's important to take reactions to the material on offer into account, as well as levels of inflammation, any dysbiosis and your pelvic tone (when thinking about insertables). Whatever you choose has to be guided not only by your physical response to the product, but your own preference as well.

Some considerations on hormonal birth control

Anything that impacts on the hormones and cycle of a fertile-age female-bodied person may have an impact on vaginal health. As we have seen, *Lactobacilli*, which reign over the vaginal microbiome, are determined and impacted upon by oestrogen. Both endogenous oestrogen (which means made in the body) or exogenous oestrogen (which means made externally to the body, such as lab-created hormones) will have an impact.

Hormonal contraception can therefore impact vaginal health. It can take the form of the combined pill, progesterone only pill, the contraceptive implant, the contraceptive injection, the contraceptive patch, the vaginal ring and intrauterine system (IUS). All of these methods use progesterone and/or oestrogen. Please refer to the NHS website to find out more about the properties of each.

When you take hormonal contraception, its effects are such that it 'takes over' from your endogenous hormones. This is why conventional medicine often uses it to attempt to control a number of hormonally-based conditions (without addressing the root cause). Based on what we have learned so far, our vaginal health is to some extent determined by our oestrogen levels, affecting our vaginal secretions and vaginal glycogen levels, which then influence our *Lactobacilli* and yeast balances. Too much oestrogen in your system might just tip you over into a thrush outbreak, and too little might make conditions optimal for BV. I'm not saying it will, but it might—and it's useful to consider this when choosing your contraception.

For the sake of completeness, it's also worth knowing that testosterone has an impact on the vulval and vaginal tissue. Normal levels of free testosterone in females are needed for a healthy vestibule area, and higher or lower levels can cause the mucosa to become thinner and feel greater levels of pain.[9]

The emotional component to vaginal health

One day I would like to conduct some research around this, because currently, in my opinion, this information is woefully missing. Through my personal experience and as a clinician, and that of my peers working in the same arena, there is an observation of an emotional component existing around vaginal health. This is a chicken-and-egg type situation. Does an emotion feed into a burgeoning infection, or does having an infection or repeated infection give us an emotional response, or, as is most likely in my opinion, both.

I don't feel inclined to be prescriptive here and list the emotions that I have noticed in both myself and the women I have helped in relation to the conditions faced, or indicate some of the emotions that lie at the root of recurring situations. Instead, I would say that if you are someone who notices you are suffering from recurring conditions vaginally, as well as trying some of the suggestions in Part Four of this book, it might be insightful to journal around what feelings they bring up for you and about your relationship to your sexual self too. I've included some journal prompts later in Part Four under Other lifestyle considerations (p. 169).

Trauma

And with that in mind, we approach the topic of trauma. Trauma can be defined as a deeply distressing or disturbing experience that we are unable to process at the time, that can be singular in nature or a series of events. That experience or experiences can be sexual, emotional, mental or physical in nature and can happen at any point on the journey of life. It can even occur during giving birth. Trauma is a complex topic and somewhat outside the scope of this book and my professional expertise. However, it is worth saying that trauma of any kind has an immense effect on the nervous system, our feelings, our perceptions, as well as our mental health, and most definitely on our emotional health. Even singular incidents can result in PTSD.

The effects it has on our nervous system and emotional health can affect our somatic health via stress held in the body through tension and tightening of the muscles (see Resources section for the work of Dr Gabor Maté). As we have seen above all of this can play into and may affect our vaginal health, as can be seen with vaginismus.

If you feel that this is relevant for you, I recommend that you seek therapy from a suitably qualified and experienced somatic, sexual or psychotherapeutic therapist. Some of the relevant professional bodies for practitioners are listed in the Resources section. It may also be worth noting that you may need to try a variety of therapists or talking therapies until you find the one that resonates with you—don't be disheartened—it's all part of the journey that serves you.

The neo-vagina and penetrative sex

As discussed previously, penetrative sex may be possible and desirable for those with a neo-vagina. Depth and girth of the neo-vagina may cause issues for intercourse, and dilators are a first-line preventative intervention to facilitate this. Surgery may also be offered as an option if necessary.

There has been some research carried out around the sexual satiety and satisfaction for those with neo-vaginas, and it remains uncertain as to whether they will be able to experience genital arousal and orgasm. In one long-term study of 19 patients who have undergone surgery to create a neo-vagina using sigmoid intestinal tissue, 16 were reported to be able to reach orgasm.[24]

Another study from 2016 showed that improved sexual innervation of the neo-vagina through a new surgical technique that created an arousal area on the anterior wall and clitoral tissue led to the generation of what the paper describes as 'adequate sexual functionality', which one could take to mean arousal, if not actual ability to orgasm.[25] This is promising in that it highlights the focus on foregrounding pleasure through functionality, as well as cosmetic changes. I consider this a major recognition of the importance of pleasure.

Peri-menopause into menopause

While many of the conditions explored in the biologically fertile years section can also occur into menopause and beyond, this section focuses on those that are more likely to arise in this life stage. The peri-menopause is defined as the years leading up to your last period, whereas menopause is a more singular event, defined technically as one year after the last day of your last period. In society we think about women as being menopausal and this is slightly confusing as the events and symptoms leading up to your last period are actually peri-menopause.

As the female body ages, it moves naturally from being considered biologically 'fertile' and having periods with the possibility of producing offspring, to no longer having periods or being biologically able to reproduce. This is part of the natural ageing process and is predominantly mediated by the reduction of the most potent form of endogenous oestrogen, oestradiol (E2), which is produced predominantly by the ovaries.

Overall, there are three main types of oestrogen produced by the body: Oestradiol (E2)—as covered above—this is also the type of oestrogen that men produce in their adrenals and testes; Oestriol (E3)—the main oestrogen in pregnancy, mainly produced by the placenta; and Oestrone (E1)—produced by adrenal glands and fatty tissue—this is the main type of circulating oestrogen post-menopause. Oestetrol (E4) is a further type of oestrogen, but is only produced during pregnancy.

All types of oestrogen affect tissues throughout the body, including regulating the menstrual cycle, and binding to receptor sites in the vagina, uterus, urinary tract, heart and blood vessels, bones, breasts, skin, hair, mucous membranes, pelvic muscles and the brain. No wonder so many effects are felt throughout the body around the menopause.

During peri-menopause, which can start as early as 40 and last for somewhere between 7 to 14 years, a variety of symptoms may become apparent. These are wide-ranging and include the classic symptoms of hot flushes, interrupted sleep and brain fog. While the average age for menopause in the Western world is 51,[26] surgical menopause due to hysterectomy, oophorectomy, mastectomy, or cancer treatment can cause peri-menopause and the cessation of periods much more abruptly at a younger age, which can be both disturbing and disruptive.

Before I move on to focusing on vaginal changes caused by declining levels of Oestrodiol during peri-menopause and menopause, and the vaginal health issues specific for that phase of life, I want to briefly mention hormone replacement therapy or HRT. Some women swear by HRT as a way of staving off the effects caused by dropping endogenous oestrogen levels. Some women wouldn't touch it with a barge pole on principle, and some are more cautious due to the perceived health risks. I'm not going to be giving a judgement call or advice on this—every woman should make her own decision about taking HRT, and part of this decision will be informed by how severe symptoms are for her. Like everything related to being human, we are all individual, with broad similarities in how our biology, psychology, etc. functions, but every woman will experience peri-menopause and menopause differently. What I can recommend, is that you do your research to enable you to reach the best decision for you.

Menopause into post-menopausal

As previously mentioned, menopause is the singular event marking one year since the last day of your last period. However, in reality this whole period is a transformational time, which can be gradual and erratic and, of course, different for every woman. Often beset with negative press around hot flushes, disrupted sleep and poor memory, it's been given a bad reputation, in line with other times in a woman's life that we've been taught to loathe (shark week anyone?!). However, let's not pathologise this stage of a woman's life. It's a perfectly natural thing to occur, and it's important to know that it doesn't *need* medicating, no matter what the dominant culture tells us. Personal choice is paramount here (and sometimes difficult to separate from the messaging we've been exposed to), and rationalising the ratio of risk-to-benefit should inform your decision making around HRT.

Instead, let's think about this time as women stepping fully into their power following the apprenticeship of their cycling years (this idea has been adopted and, I suppose, endorsed by inclusion, from the book Wild Power by Alexandra Pope and Sjanie Hugo Wurlitzer). How does that land with you?

Re-focusing back onto vaginal health, here's some considerations for this stage of life:

Vaginal changes and what to expect

Dropping oestrogen levels are responsible for so many changes in our body around this phase of life. One of oestrogen's functions is that it 'plumps' tissue. Tissues that have the most oestrogen receptors are the most affected by this. When levels fall, so does that plumping effect. One of the outcomes of this is that the vagina, over which our natural oestrogen exerts a large effect, may atrophy, to a greater or lesser extent depending on the individual. This will happen on a cellular level which then affects the whole structure of the vagina.

One of the most obvious effects of this is that the vagina loses some of its flexibility and ability to lubricate. This may present as vaginismus and could impact intercourse depending on its extent: It can affect day-to-day to day comfort, causing the feeling of irritation in the vagina and vulva. I've worked with clients who have reported a range of sensations from little to no effect, to feeling like there are shards of broken glass stabbing the inside of their vagina if intercourse is attempted (remember that rich nerve network down there).

However, help is at hand, and I have a colleague who has passed through menopause who likes to refer to the post-menopausal vagina as a desert flower. Therapeutically, assistance may come from lubricants (as above, I've been told that a combination of water-based and oil-based ones provides that little extra, depending on whether barrier methods are being used); vaginal moisturisers, which are very similar to lubricants but used on a daily comfort basis and applied using applicators; and topical HRT creams which can be very helpful if the 'shards-of-glass' feeling is what's going on for you.

Using HRT topically has a lower set of health risks when compared with systemic HRT use. There is also some promising preliminary research on pelvic muscle floor training as well as nasal breathing exercises for dryness and atrophy, and this is an area worth keeping an eye on and possibly exploring with a female pelvic health physio.[27, 27a] Also, see the sections on 'fennel', 'pessaries', the therapeutics listed under 'hormonal' and 'sea buckthorn oil' in the Therapeutics section coming up next.

My dear vagina
You have served me well
You traded for clothes and meals
You have negotiated some very good deals

You have been active since we turned 16
Back then you were moist, elastic, pristine

When we reached 45 you began to wince
Even if we were trading with our favourite dream prince
You began to dry, become tight and sore
Vitamin E pessaries became a regular product in the drawer

After a while, these weren't enough
And off to the sexual health clinic, we adjourned

Localised HRT and extra lube came next
Which was such a relief from what had become
Such painful sex

So now, twice a week, an applicator you must endure
Thank you and I love you little vagina
To my very, very core ♥

—Claire A. Lodge

Changes in the microbiome

We already know that our vaginal microbiome relies on oestrogen to produce glycogen-rich mucous to feed the *Lactobacilli*, which keeps the vaginal ecology in good health. With falling natural oestrogen levels, less natural lubrication and glycogen-rich mucous is produced, meaning that, in many cases, the *Lactobacilli* population reduces. In a lower oestrogen/*Lactobacilli* environment the bacteria responsible for bacterial vaginosis (BV) are much more likely to proliferate without the check of the *Lactobacilli*, and this can be a problem for some people. In fact, BV-causing bacteria and BV itself are much more likely to be a cause of infection than *Candida* spp., which prefer an oestrogen- and glycogen-rich environment to grow. This is worth bearing in mind when looking for likely culprits for infection during this life stage.

In recent years, HRT use has gone some way to reduce that trend, but with the outcome of more post-menopausal women experiencing thrush than would naturally.

Freedom and power

In traditional ways of looking at the earth, humans and the seasons, the three ages of womanhood are commonly known as Maiden, Mother and Crone. You may have heard of this yourself. If you have, what do you think of it? I've always wondered how I personally connected to these three identities. Maiden, sure (twirls my long strawberry blonde hair). Mother, maybe. Crone, just … urgh. Although this triad is known and used widely in more esoteric circles in the Western/English speaking world, I believe it is also more subtly woven into our wider culture, sitting alongside other ways we have for identifying the roles women play (think of the whore/madonna dichotomy here in particular). Society is happy to sexualise the Maiden, revere the Mother, but what about the Crone? It conjures all sorts of negative associations. We may visualise a woman—old, withered, haggard, ugly, ostracised and possibly feared—the witch figure of cartoons and fairy tales. The Crone symbolises that third age of woman, once she has passed through the menopause, and gone beyond her sexually fertile age. In dominant culture we rarely see this female archetype as positive, powerful, wise and knowledgeable. Why is that?

Leaving that question dangling in the air (I don't want to be as crass as to name the reason—but we all know right?*), and because Crone can so easily conjure negative mental images, I propose rather to adopt the term Mage instead, that I saw a good friend and fellow herbalist Amaia Dadachanji use recently. So what does Mage conjure for you instead? What meaning is held in that name instead? Does it feel more powerful and more positive? Something to be revered? A power to attain and hold? To me that feels more exciting and, most importantly, more accurate.

I've not yet reached the Mage stage, but from those I know around me, I see amazing women with many years' experience and knowledge who have honed and learned their gifts. To be valued for this, and as being the matriarch in community groups; the grandmother figure who helps to raise the next generation; passing wisdom on; or those at the top of their game in their profession; holding positions of authority: Society should be supporting these women's role in the community and workplace. To do anything other is to blindly marginalise a lifetime of knowledge and feminine knowledge. How does it feel to embrace this idea of Mage?

Another important topic that we should cover around this life stage is that of sexual freedom! Menstruation and the possibility of producing offspring has finished, and the issue of 'family planning' is no longer an issue in sexual concerns. Barrier methods of contraception that may once have been used are often forgone. This may feel freeing and the sense of feminine sexual freedom and agency should be celebrated. However, a reduction in the use of barrier methods due to lack of concerns about pregnancy has seen a rise in STIs in the over 65s, of a greater proportional increase than any other age group in the UK in 2019![28]

With this in mind remember to use condoms or another barrier method, even post-menopausally. Not using a barrier method also has a direct impact on the vaginal microbiome because a partner's intimate microbiome will be introduced to the area, possibly affecting and influencing the environment.

Suggested treatments: Therapeutics in the Hormonal (p. 151) and pH modulation (p. 153) sections would be helpful during this transition time.

*the answer is the patriarchy

Talking to partners about vaginal health

We have covered the concerns of women regarding our vaginal health. But let's not forget the people of other genders in this equation. Our partners, friends, sons, fathers, brothers and community members. Their advocacy and understanding can be *so* important in how we show up in the world when our vaginas aren't functioning in the way we would like.

Traditionally a difficult subject for women to verbalise and vocalise, it has also been a tricky subject for men to hear about or bear witness to. A history of silence has compounded this. It has contributed to feelings of shame, alienation, guilt, isolation and discomfort—felt on both sides of the conversation that, so often, you're not having. Vaginal health— that icky topic …

Hopefully, we are at a frontier where we can start to change that. Let's be the change. And that starts at home. Every voice is important in this mission. Don't think that it doesn't matter if you speak up or not. It does. So how can we have healthy and helpful communication around vaginal health with our nearest and dearest other, especially if the vagina is stigmatised as a sexual object through society's lens? What benefits can we as individuals and as society enjoy if we do?

Well, firstly, we will have an ease of communication which affords intimacy, clarity and understanding. Then we help pioneer a new era where we shred the shame around vaginal health and can have open and useful conversations about our bodies.

I invited my friend and colleague Andrea Balboni, the sex, love and relationships coach to share some of the recommendations she uses with clients in how to initiate these conversations. Here is what she has to say:

> It can feel exceptionally challenging to open up a conversation with our partners about a part of our bodies that many of us aren't used to fully acknowledging. Even to ourselves. You may feel that you yourself are just beginning to connect with your body and know it in a way that you never have before. This new intimate connection with yourself can feel quite tender and delicate, like most new relationships.
>
> And it can take a while to put language that feels natural, empowering and good to parts of ourselves that we've often been taught are shameful or should not be mentioned to anyone—not even ourselves. We tend to fall back on phrases like 'down there' or 'downstairs', as if naming a body part for what it is somehow wrong or shameful.
>
> And while vulva or vagina may be difficult to mention, it is more the embarrassment we've been taught to feel around our bodies that is what is difficult to manage. As you build an intimate relationship with yourself and begin to accept your body— all parts of you—as beautiful and natural, then conversation will feel easier with your partner. In the meantime, here are some ways that you can initiate a conversation around the health of your body, and in particular that most sacred and beautiful part of you, your vagina, with your partner.

Invite the conversation and agree on a time:

- I'd like to have a conversation about what is happening with my body, is there a good time today?
  If you say 'Can you talk now?', then you activate defence mechanisms. Try asking:
- Is now a good time to have a conversation about this?
  Create safety: Name the elephant in the room.
- It is difficult and challenging for me to speak about this. And I suspect it might be for you as well. However, it's important for me to share this with you. And I'd love to learn how you feel about it.
  Let the other person know that neither of you will be judged. And that open honest questions are welcome.
  Have the conversation outside of the bedroom. By taking the conversation out of the context of the bedroom, it can feel as if there is more space for open communication. A more neutral environment can facilitate an easier exchange of feelings and thoughts.
  Preparing yourself for the conversation:

- Journaling practice: fears, clearings, desires.
- Let go of your fears, gather your thoughts and clear your mind by doing this simple free-writing exercise before you meet your partner.
- Write whatever comes to mind. Don't think about it. Just let whatever wants to come, flow onto the paper.

Journal prompt 1:
What do you fear about having a conversation with your partner about vaginal health?
Examples:

- I fear that I'll feel embarrassed and so will he. That it will be awkward and weird.
- I fear that by naming what is going on with me that he'll reject me and my body.
- I fear that I'll not be able to say what I need to say.

Journal prompt 2:
What do you clear about having the conversation?

- I clear the fear that I have.
- I clear the shame I feel around talking about my body.
- I clear how alone I've felt by not being able to share up until now.

Journal prompt 3:
What do you desire as a result of having the conversation?

- I desire to be seen and understood.
- I desire support around what I'm going through.
- I desire to be loved and accepted as I am.

Sharing with your partner in this way can feel very vulnerable. Know that it is by being vulnerable with one another, that we come closer together.

You can find more about Andrea's work in the Resources section (p. 192).

PART FOUR

THERAPEUTICS

We've looked at the vast majority of issues that affect vaginas of all ages, throughout life. I tell you, it was something to write, at times confronting and heavy, but we got there. We've made it and now here's what I (and most herbalists) think of as the fun part: Therapeutics! By that I mean, what we can do therapeutically to help ourselves at home. Yes!!!! Roll up your sleeves and get prepared to take back some control, get your hands the best kind of 'dirty' and have some fun.

We start with a look at all the different dosage forms—that is, all the ways you can take and use natural remedies—then we move on to the Materia Medica, which covers the natural agents we may consider using (the herbs and supplements if you will). We will also look at lifestyle interventions.

But firstly, a word about when to get professional help. Everything contained in this section is designed to give you some power over your own vaginal health. Herbal and holistic health generally looks at root causes, as well as symptomatic relief, rather than just symptomatic relief alone.

Limitations

It's important to realise the limitations of what you can work with and achieve by yourself. In general, if what you are trying to resolve has:

- Been going on for longer than a cycle or two
- You have blood-stained discharge or breakthrough bleeding
- Is a recurring issue that isn't getting better
- Symptoms of fever or unexplained weight loss
- Pain on intercourse
- Pain on urination with vaginal discharge or a history of this
- If you suspect you have an STI
- You are in unbearable discomfort
- If something alarms you
- You don't have a clear diagnosis
- Something happens that's unusual for you and your body
- You have another condition or illness
- You are on other pharmaceutical medicines
- You are, or might be, pregnant.

Then you need to seek professional help in the form of a qualified practitioner, such as a herbalist or naturopath who specialises in this area and is registered with a professional body, or your GP. (NB I'm really supportive of GPs and the NHS in general—they have amazing diagnostic tools, lifesaving medicine and some of their therapeutics can be very helpful indeed and definitely have their place!).

It's also important to note that just because something is 'natural' it doesn't automatically mean that it's safe. Some of nature's strongest poisons are from plants. Respect natural medicine, follow the safety advice, warnings and dosages and if in doubt, don't feel afraid to seek professional help. If you haven't said 'yes' to anything on the above list, then you are clear to go ahead and select remedies that might be appropriate for you.

Questions to ask yourself

The following questions may help you when choosing your herbs:

- Is the problem acute (recently flared up) or chronic (a longer-term problem that can often exist in the background with occasional flare-ups)—if chronic or longer-term, then you should definitely consider a whole-body approach.
- Are you in immediate discomfort? Then you should address this in any first approach you take, as well as looking holistically at your health.
- Did you answer yes to any of the questions on the Limitations list? Please go to see a practitioner.

Dosage forms

This is a term used in traditional Western herbal medicine (the form of herbal medicine that I practice that combines science and tradition) to refer to the medicinal formats that herbs are used in. If you think about it, unless you are prepared to ingest sufficient quantities of fresh herb material from a source you trust (and bear in mind that some of the herbs you might want to use aren't growing in your proverbial back garden) it seems pretty sensible to find ways that you can manage to preserve, concentrate and take the herbs you want to get therapeutic benefit from. This doesn't necessarily mean you need to take loads of a herb for it to do its thing—some can and do work in a very subtle, energetic way.

In this section, I outline some of the most common dosage forms you're going to encounter as you dive into natural healing. These are practical ways for you to take your herbs. As you do, bear in mind that medicinal plants are a complex synergy of many hundreds of naturally occurring phyto (plant)—chemicals. In allopathic (pharmaceutical) medicine we are used to single compounds being isolated for use in a medicine. Plants work differently to that. Whereas in pharmaceutical medicine we readily accept unwanted effects alongside the desired outcomes, in many cases the complex chemistry of a medicinal plant has an amphoteric effect, balancing out some of the unwanted effects, and instead interacting with the dynamic body it finds itself ingested by.

The majority of the phytochemicals found in plants are either water soluble or lipid (fats)/alcohol soluble. Such is the nature of chemistry. The different dosage forms exploit this fact. If you choose to use fresh plant material (that you may have foraged yourself) be sure of identification, only pick what nature can afford to spare you (i.e. don't strip out any habitat and always leave enough for the animals), always pick above dog height and away from polluted areas, and remember that fresh plant material has a higher water content. This means you will need more material than if you were using a dried form to make the equivalent strength, although it might make energetically more vibrant medicine.

Tea and decoctions

Teas or tisanes are the simplest water extractions you can prepare using a herb. Most are made to be drunk and are classed as internal medicines. The vast majority are made by pouring boiling water on herb material (1 oz to 1 pint: 30 g to 600 ml[29]) and left to steep for 5–10 minutes before draining and using. They can also be used in making topical preparations such as creams or sitz baths (see below).

Decoctions are also water extracts, used for the same purpose, but are made by boiling the herb material in the water for around ten minutes. This is most useful for root, bark or dried fruit material. It gains the maximum water extraction but does break down some of the compounds that we may be wanting to use, such as polysaccharides. Chemistry again!

In some cases, cold water infusions are best for the chemistry of the plant we are using—I will indicate further on if any herbs are better extracted using this method. One point to note is that water preparations do not preserve well and even if kept in the fridge need to be used within a day of making.

Tincture

Simply put, a tincture is an alcoholic extraction of a herb. The way that most tinctures are made mean that water is also used, meaning that both the water-soluble and the alcohol/lipid-soluble phytochemical are extracted into the resulting tincture. Again, most tinctures are made to be drunk and are classed as internal medicines, although sometimes they are used in the making of external preparations like creams. Due to the use of high percentage alcohol, tinctures last much, much longer than teas, and when used in external preparations can exert a drying effect on the area—this won't be ideal for topical use on vulval and vaginal tissue.

Tinctures can be made at home, but most often they can be easily purchased from suppliers such as Neals Yard Remedies, Baldwins, Dee Atkinson, Botanica Medica and Apotheca Natural Health (other places do exist too! See Resources p. 189). On the labels of the bottles you buy you will see the alcoholic strength of the tincture by percentage, as well as a ratio. This ratio will tell you how much herb material (marc) was used to alcohol (menstruum). Ergo, a 1:3 tincture means one part herb to three parts alcohol. The marc can be made up of dried or fresh plant material, but remember to take into account the higher water content in fresh plants, meaning that the strength of the tincture will be slightly less than if you used its dried equivalent by weight.

Tinctures are taken internally—normally in a little water before food (otherwise the taste is too strong). The dosage varies depending on what it is, why you are taking it and whether it is a simple (a tincture made from one herb) or a mix of tinctures. Due to the alcoholic nature of tinctures, they may not be suitable for you on certain religious grounds, if you have liver disease or problems with alcohol addiction.

Information on the dosage of each herb is included in each entry.

Sitz bath and washes

Sitz baths are water preparations of herbs, used externally in a hip bath. Simples (a single herb) can be used, but it is more normal for combinations of herbs to be used. Herbs are made into a tea, as above, then allowed to cool to a temperature that would be suitable to bathe in. The herbs are then strained off (or made in a 'tea bag'—a foot from a pair of tights, tied off, is perfect for this) and the resultant 'tea' is then placed in the hip bath—enough liquid is needed to cover the hips. You then sit in the bath and relax while the herbs do their thing.

While I don't recommend using distilled essential oils topically for vaginal and vulval issues, even when mixed with something else, tiny amounts of essential oils that are naturally present in a plant do come out in teas. Often they are carried away on the steam, but some may remain suspended in the water infusion, and in this form they may be useful therapeutically.

Hip baths can be quite hard to source these days and I often advocate using a large, clean washing up bowl or a shallow full-sized bath, if you have one at home. The important thing is that there is enough room and 'tea' to cover your hips and reach your intimate areas.

Sitz baths are fabulous for vaginal and vulval conditions as you are allowing the herbs to get full external contact with the areas they are aiming to reach. They can be used daily while in an acute phase and are useful for post-birth healing. It's important to check there are no open wounds before exposing the area to a sitz bath, however.

Compresses

Compresses are herbs applied to an area using a cloth. They can either be made of water preparations of herbs, or use fresh plants. For a water-based preparation, make a strong tea from dried herbs and when cool, soak a cloth with it and apply directly to an area of the body. If fresh herbs are used, crush them to break open the plant cells and place them in a cloth, before applying it directly to the area in question.

I always advocate the use of organic muslin for a compress, both for the quality and assurance of the material, but also it's porous nature. I love using compresses for inflammation where I want to ensure a good, cooling application of herbs but where I do not want any extraneous material left behind, any excipients, or where it is not convenient or practical to use a sitz bath.

Steams

Although having gained some mixed reviews in the mainstream press in the last couple of years, I can assure you vaginal steaming is not for cosmetic purposes. Vaginal steaming is about vaginal and female health, and most women who do it say that it is deeply nourishing, relaxing and releasing. Using herbal steams in this way can be wonderfully healing and nourishing for numerous female symptoms, bringing blood flow to the area for healing and imparting the benefits of essential oils in a very gentle way. It is a traditional form of female healing originating in a variety of indigenous cultures around the world.

You will need your herb mix, boiling water, a bowl, a towel, 20 minutes of undisturbed alone time and a toilet, a steaming stool with slats or holes, plus two large handfuls of fresh herbs; if you are using dried herbs, just one generous handful. Boil a large pan of water and then pour into the bowl you will use for the steam. Let it cool for a few minutes off the boil so that it does not burn your skin, then add the herbs. Place in the toilet bowl, or on the floor under the steaming stool.

Take your underwear off, but make sure you wear socks. Sit on the chair, draping a heavy towel or a blanket around your waist to trap the steam in. Be careful not to allow any drafts in, so make sure the blanket covers you and reaches to the floor. Don't get cold from the waist up either!

Remain sitting over the steam for 20 minutes. This is a good time for meditation, reading or simply to sit quietly and enjoy the herbal healing. The heat should feel pleasant. If it is too warm, wait for a few minutes and try again. *Do not burn yourself!*

Rest quietly after the herbal steam in a warm room free from drafts or open windows. It is best to go to bed for at least an hour. Be careful for the next 24 hours to protect yourself from cold drafts, keep warm and avoid sudden temperature changes. If you are trying to conceive and are not taking contraception, only steam before you ovulate. Do not steam if there is any chance that you may be pregnant, have an IUD fitted or have a gynaecological cancer.

Pessaries

You've probably heard of pessaries, if not used them yourself. Different from suppositories (which are bigger and designed for rectal application, that is, up the bum, and not necessarily related to vaginal health), these have an active ingredient, in our case plant extracts. These are combined with excipients. In our case we can use natural excipients, which may also confer vaginally-healing properties, into small (normally 1–2 g by total weight per pessary) bullet-shaped masses, that are useful for vaginal insertion.

Great for getting the therapeutic agents to where they need to be for a number of hours, pessaries are most commonly used overnight. They are inserted with a clean finger, high into your vagina before bed (but all the way to the cervix is not necessary), and allowed to 'melt' due to body heat (only ever insert one per night). Often oily in composition, it's recommended that you wear a pad on the nights you use a pessary, and often the following day too, to avoid ruining underwear (don't use your best pants either, just in case).

Unlike many pharmaceutical pessaries, herbal pessaries are applied consecutively over 5–7 nights at a time. You can make them yourself if you are clear which is the best type to make for your situation, and if you have something you can fashion into or use as, a mould (some of the silicone chocolate or ice cube moulds may work for this, depending on shape) and should be kept in the fridge to preserve their shape and prevent them from melting.

A typical recipe for a commonly prescribed oil-based pessary would be 20 g of a solid base oil such as Cocoa butter to 10 ml of infused oil, which are then gently heated together and mixed when the solid oil has melted and then poured into a pessary mould and allowed to set.

The vagina is not a pocket

I heard this great phrase from my fellow practitioners at Invivo Healthcare, and it's a brilliant reminder that the vagina is not an experimental playground. If you do decide to make your own pessaries or insert products internally, it's good to remember this and only select herbs you know to be safe for you and that will nourish your microbiome. Traditionally, essential oils such as tea tree have been used to make pessaries to clear vaginal thrush. I would question the use of such a direct application of essential oils—as they are likely to kill good bacteria as well as target fungal or bacterial overgrowth—and it would be best to work with a knowledgeable practitioner if this is the way you wanted to go, so you could preserve your vaginal microbiome. Also, be mindful of the pH of the overall mix of ingredients. Where the vagina is concerned, pH reigns supreme!

At this point I'd like to tell you a little story of a client I was working with a few years ago. Before starting to work with me, she had been unsure what was going on for her and had been googling things to help the conditions she believed she may have been suffering from. One night, in utter desperation, she first tried inserting one remedy that was strongly acidic in nature into her vagina, and then when that hadn't alleviated any of the symptoms within an hour or two, she inserted a remedy that was strongly alkaline. In classic chemistry style, the reaction inside her vagina produced heat and water, and she ended up messaging me in the small hours from A&E wanting advice to not only get to the root of the problem but help soothe her poor inflamed vagina. The message from this story is that when working topically with the vagina, be sure of what specific condition you wish to treat, diagnose it via testing, and then try one thing at a time to avoid any adverse reactions.

Other topical preparations—cream, ointments and gels

There may be times when other topical preparations might be useful for your vaginal and vulval health. Creams and Ointments both have an oil component which makes them incompatible with barrier methods of contraception.

Ointments can be useful if you want to create a barrier for the skin while applying the herbs (nappy rash might be one of these times, for example). Cream-making has a water phase as well as an oil phase, and requires a method of preservation to stop the growth of bacteria. Having a water phase means that creams are lighter than ointments, are more readily absorbed into the skin and also have a pH (only water-based substances have a pH).

pH is worth bearing in mind when thinking about which topical application you might want to use for the vagina or vulva.

Other factors to consider are whether the ingredients you use in your preparation will impact or kill the vaginal microbiome, whether the excipients have a heating or cooling effect, and what this would be like for the condition you are treating. Oils in general have a heating effect as they 'trap' any heat into the skin. Gels on the other hand are more cooling in nature. Gels such as aloe vera are water-based and mucilaginous, meaning that they hold their form and can be a very soothing way to apply herbs to intimate areas.

Abdominal massage

When I first trained in abdominal massage, my then work colleagues got a bit confused and thought that I'd trained in vaginal massage—when I arrived back in the office I had to correct them—no siree, that's not what I do (but it is a thing and is advocated by wonderful folk like Layla Martin for increased connection to your sexual energy, but it's not what I do!).

Abdominal massage is a traditional female health practice in many cultures around the world. Best known in the UK as Mayan abdominal massage, it may also be called (with subtle differences) Arvigo massage, womb massage, fertility massage and Mizan massage. Focused on the abdominal area, the back and sometimes the legs, it helps stimulate the circulatory and eliminatory pathways and organs, including the digestive system, connective tissue and lymphatic system, as well as the pelvic and reproductive organs, to help clear pelvic congestion, and increase vitality in the area. It doesn't involve touching intimate areas (but it does involve massaging the stomach) and can be helpful for conditions that may benefit from reducing any sense of pelvic congestion, such as thrush and prolapse, along with other gynaecological conditions. Please note it may not be suitable if you are in the first trimester of pregnancy, may be pregnant, or you have an IUD fitted.

Once you have seen a therapist for the first time, and they have taken a full case history and performed the massage, you will also be taught self-massage techniques to be used at home as a top-up and maintenance in-between your sessions. If you are interested to learn more, please see the Resources section in Part Five where there are links to various organisations that can put you in a touch with a practitioner (p. 189).

What do I mean when I talk about energetics?

As you may have gathered by now, and what you will notice as we wander into the Materia Medica section (the section that talks about the medicinal plant material), is that I sometimes talk about energy or energetics. This is a key component of natural medicine and something that is simply missing from many aspects of pharmaceutical health care and modern life today.

When I talk about energy in this way, or energetics as a whole, I am referring to the quality of life-force of a particular plant, or perhaps a person or type of condition too. The best way to illustrate this is by looking at Eeyore and Winnie the Pooh from the classic A. A. Milne stories. Just from looking at them we can tell that Winnie the Pooh has a cheerful, sunny disposition and Eeyore is more depressed and pessimistic. As we hear them speak and see how they act, this characterisation is further confirmed and we develop a vocabulary to describe each of them distinctly. From this example, we can see that we all intrinsically have an understanding of what energetics means. Just like the characters in the Milne stories, plant species have a set of energetic characteristics too, that we can understand and describe when we get to know a plant.

Understanding the energetics of a plant may tell us something about how they interact in the body too. This is in addition to their pharmacological actions in the body—their energy interacts with our energy as well as the energetics of the conditions we may be experiencing. A traditional way to start putting words to the energetics of plants, people and conditions is through the cardinal points of heat, cold, wet and dry. We may understand in a simplistic way that thrush is a hot, wet condition. We can then understand that we are looking for a remedy that might be energetically cooling and drying.

As we move into the Materia Medica section below, we will discover the energetic character of these plants and how they may interact with the body at this level, which may lead to clues about how they might best be used.

Sex

A word on intercourse while you are treating a vaginal or vulval infection. In general, I advise my patients to abstain from intercourse during this time, and also to treat their partner/s for the same thing too, if it is an infection of some kind. This is because you don't want to keep passing whatever is going on back and forth between you. Intercourse may also increase irritation for you due to friction and micro-trauma to the tissues. While I understand that it can be hard to agree on abstaining from penetration for the duration, I really do recommend it. It can be helpful to refer to the section above on talking to partners about vaginal health for how to communicate to your partner around this, and to think up other ways to be intimate during this time.

Materia Medica

How to use this section and how to choose your remedies

When you head to the internet for advice on home or natural remedies, sometimes they might work for you and sometimes they might not. It can be hit and miss for vaginal health (or any health condition for that matter). Sometimes that might be because you have something other than what you thought and the treatment you're trying isn't the right one, or can be that through trying one or two things in quick succession your body isn't getting the additional support it needs to make treatment a success. Sometimes the internet isn't specific enough. It treats natural remedies as one-hit wonders, the way we pop pharmaceutical pills—a one-stop wonder-bullet to get rid of troublesome symptoms.

My colleagues and I work holistically and that's how I want you to approach your health too. That means we're not just treating a site on the body, a symptom, an organism (though we are doing that too) with the natural version of a pharmaceutical wonder-pill (that may or may not work for you), but we're also supporting the whole of you so that your body can keep your vaginal health in homeostasis ensuring that when you clear something up, it, or something else, doesn't come back.

Materia Medica is an old Latin medical term meaning the knowledge about a collection of therapeutic substances, and in this section, we not only get into the herbs, but other supplements and lifestyle interventions that can be useful when dealing with vaginal health conditions. In Part Three of this book I have recommended some approaches and aims for different conditions where appropriate, and these are great specifics to look at when taking charge of your vaginal health.

This section is divided into broad categories that we can use to describe the Materia Medica contained within. In herbal medicine, these aren't hard and fast reductionist delineations, but rather groupings that can help us understand some of the actions of the therapeutics mentioned. Many plants, or indeed supplements, may in fact demonstrate action in several categories listed, or even categories we are not concerned with here. It's a broader scheme.

When listing the herbs, I have approached them in a similar way to how they would appear in a traditional herbal, including the best dosage form to use it in. Where a herb has already been covered in a different section, I list it again to let you know that you would use it in this way too. When listing supplements, diet and lifestyle advice, I give information about what it is and the way to use it.

Hierarchy of therapeutics

When building a regime for yourself for your vaginal health, take care of any uncomfortable, acute symptoms first, possibly with topical applications. I would then advise a layered approach that looks at you as a whole and takes into account any lifestyle interventions required. Don't forget that testing—so you know what you have—is key here.

Layer 1
The first areas to assess are your immunity, your digestion and waste elimination. In virtually all of my patients, I need to start here as the basis for helping them.

Layer 2
Nervous system support is crucial as nerve pain, stress and mental health can come into play when looking at vaginal health. Nervines are also where the aphrodisiacs sit. Nervous system support will underpin any work you do to reduce symptoms and clear up the issue.

Layer 3
Consider whether inflammation is an issue for you—if so, explore the suggestions for anti-inflammatory therapeutics. If it is, you may wish to include some support for your vaginal mucous membranes from the Mucous Membrane section. Irritation and inflammation often needs to be calmed down before you go in with any of the topical applications that clear up the problem.

Layer 4
Then comes the specific recommendations in the aims and approaches for each condition. Don't overcomplicate it for yourself. When choosing the herbs, consider whether you are going to use them topically (i.e. on the vulval skin or in the vagina) or take them orally. If you are taking them orally, decide whether you will take them as tinctures or

dried herbs. Once you have decided on the herbs that are right for you, it's fine to take them all together in a tea or as a combined tincture. You might even find one herb covers two areas—that often happens in herbal medicine and is one of the super cool things about it.

I recommend that you stick to no more than five herbs at a time, and a handful of supplements, dietary changes and lifestyle interventions. Any more and it can become overwhelming to manage, and not everything in that mix may suit you. Also, remember, the vagina is not a pocket (see above—this is important!). Do all of this with a mind to the limitations set out in the section above. If any of those come into play, it's time to see a professional! Make that promise to me and to yourself.

How long to stay on the herbs and when to retake

In terms of self-treatment at home, unless your symptoms get worse, allow yourself four weeks to see improvement. Any longer than that and I suggest you go to see a practitioner.

What to do when everything reacts?

In some cases, what you might use topically may react and cause an increase in your symptoms. If that happens, try to remove what you used, and bathe the area with plain water (but do not douche). A cool green tea compress or a bicarb sitz bath may be helpful, but do not keep trying different things on the area; otherwise, you might make a bad situation worse. If it doesn't calm down, it's best to book in to see a qualified practitioner who can help guide you.

Getting to know herbs

The best way to get to know a herb is to sit with it, take it and see how it feels in the body. This can be a meditative process and it's a process I really recommend using to get to know these beautiful living medicine allies. All the herbs here have been chosen due to their relative ease of access and safety. Use the guidance above and the safety notes included below, but don't experiment if you are on medication without seeing a medical herbalist or nutritional therapist.

Anti-inflammatory

Chamomile

Name: Chamomile, Roman or German *Anthemis nobilis* or *Matricaria recutita*

Also known as: Mayweed, maythen

Plant family: *Asteraceae* (daisy)

Part used: Flower heads

Known constituents: Coumarins; flavonoids in particular apigenin, apigetrin, apiin, luteolin, quercetin, quercimeritrin and rutin; volatile (essential) oils, in particular a-bisabolol and chamazulene (responsible for the blue colour sometimes detected in the tea or essential oil), amino acids, anthemic acid, choline, polysaccharides, plant acids, fatty acids, tannins and triterpene hydrocarbons.[30]

Key words: Summer; childhood; softness; mothering.

Actions: Relaxing; anti-inflammatory; anti-allergy; antimicrobial; sedative, antiviral; anti-spasmodic; mild antiseptic.

Emotional uses: Wonderful for outbursts of anger which come from a place of fear, or for when you are feeling prickly and oversensitive, chamomile brings a relaxing, centring feeling of softness, security and nourished wellbeing.[31]

Physical uses: Chamomile's anti-allergic and anti-inflammatory actions are well documented and much of this is attributed to the essential oil content.[30] While I wouldn't recommend applying the essential oil directly, when it is suspended in a water infusion it can be very useful therapeutically. A sedative effect has been documented in animal studies (aside from the ethical issue, how useful animal studies are when translating to effects in humans we cannot say), but contrary to popular culture's belief, chamomile's main use isn't really to aid sleep.

Chamomile has also been reported to have anti-fungal and antibacterial action against gram-positive bacteria.[30] Bartram reports the use of chamomile externally for inflammation of the skin and mucosa, including the oral cavity and gums, respiratory tract and anal and genital area,[32] and I would concur with that. It is also known amongst herbalists as 'mother of the gut'.

Suggested use: Although there are slight differences between them, I would say that Roman or German chamomile are interchangeable in the way that we want to use it here. External application of a water extract of chamomile is wonderful to use where intimate irritation exists and skin healing is required. It can also be helpful if allergy is part of the picture. Use as a sitz bath or make up a strong tea and use as a compress when cool enough (add in some ice cubes to cool a hot, inflamed situation). **Combines well with** marigold, green tea and/or plantain. It may be used internally as a tea to cool down any prickliness you're feeling emotionally.

Safety considerations: There is a lack of clinic safety data around chamomile, but it has been reported that those with an allergy to the daisy family may find that chamomile produces a reaction. You are likely to know if this is you. There are no documented drug interactions and, due to insufficient data, excessive use of chamomile should be avoided in pregnancy and lactation.[30]

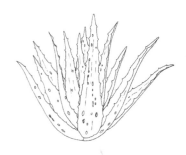

Aloe vera

Name: Aloe vera *Aloe barbadensis*

    Also known as: True aloe, first aid plant

    Plant family: *Asphodelaceae*

    Part used: Leaf juice

    Known constituents: Mono- and polysaccharides; sterols; organic acids; enzymes; saponins; vitamins; minerals and lipids.

    Key words: Cooling; moist; protective.

    Actions: Astringent; demulcent; antibacterial; mild analgesic; possible antiviral;[32] ant-arthritic; anti-inflammatory; possible anti-fungal.

    Emotional uses: I always find a great sense of physical relief when using aloe gel.

    Physical uses: Note that we are talking about the clear gel, taken from the inside of the leaf. This is distinguished from the bitter yellow juice that can be found just under the leaf's surface. This yellow juice is used as a laxative and not what we are referring to here. Aloe vera gel is well known for its use in sunburn, radiation burn and burns in general. Internally, it has been found to be useful for gastric and peptic ulcers, as well as skin ulcers, and wound healing in general.[30]

Suggested use: Because of its mucilaginous, protective, cooling nature, and the possibility that it has anti-fungal, anti-inflammatory and antibacterial properties, it is wonderfully soothing for irritated mucous membranes of the intimate areas. Use it as the base of any topical application that you intend to apply to the surface of any vulval condition where inflammation is present. **Combines well with** any other water or oil preparation used externally, such as marigold, chamomile and/or plantain.

Safety considerations: Used externally there are no documented concerns.

Witch hazel

Name: Witch hazel *Hamamelis virginiana*

Also known as: Winter bloom. Witch comes from the Old English *wice*, meaning bendable.

Plant family: *Hamamelidaceae*

Part used: Leaves, bark

Known constituents: Tannins; flavonoids; saponins; vitamin P; and a volatile oil.

Key words: Shrinking; cooling.

Actions: Haemostatic; anti-inflammatory; cleansing astringent; wound healing; styptic.[33]

Physical uses: Wonderful for bruising, sprains and strains; you might be familiar with distilled witch hazel, obtained from the chemist for facial acne. This is a distilled water extract and probably the easiest way to use this herb. It is used for mild skin injuries, local inflammation of the skin and mucous membranes, haemorrhoids (in a suppository) and itchy varicose veins. It can also be used in a liniment for aching sore muscles.[34]

Suggested use: While this could be added to a sitz bath or compress when skin healing is needed, I would recommend the main use for us here would be as a 'padsicle' mentioned in the Post Birth section, where witch hazel is sprayed onto maternity pads which are then frozen before popping into your pants to help calm and heal any perineal trauma after giving birth. **Combines well with** aloe vera.

Safety considerations: Avoid taking this herb internally, due to the intolerably high tannin content.

Green tea

Name: Green tea *Camellia sinensis*

　　Also known as: Tea plant

　　Plant family: *Theaceae*

　　Part used: Cured leaf

　　Known constituents: Caffeine; polyphenols including epigallocatechin gallate (EGCG), epicatechin gallate, epicatechins and flavanols; flavonoids including kaempferol, quercetin and myricetin; catechins; tannins.

　　Key words: Cooling; drying; stimulant.

　　Actions: Astringent; antioxidant; hypoglycaemic; cooling; anti-biofilms; anti-inflammatory; digestive.

　　Emotional uses: Reviving and stimulating, we all know how connecting and comforting a cup of tea can be.

　　Physical uses: Mostly used internally as a tea for its stimulating and antioxidant benefits, it is one of the most consumed plants on the planet. The high tannin content makes the tea quite astringent, and this can be felt in the mouth when you drink it—it feels like it's drying, or 'tightening' the inside of your mouth.

　　Suggested use: Use green tea externally, as a water extract made as a tea which is then allowed to cool. Once cool it can be used as a compress, a sitz bath or frozen onto flannels to provide relief to irritated mucous membranes. There is also some evidence that green tea used topically in this way inhibits the formation of biofilms and may in fact disrupt them. It can therefore be used in CVVC, Mollicutes and BV where biofilm formation makes it difficult for therapeutic agents to act on and clear any infection. **Combines well with** marigold, chamomile, apple cider vinegar in external applications.

　　Safety considerations: Internally, it can be overstimulating if drunk in large quantities or for those who are anxious. It can also be depleting for those with a sensitive digestive system.[35] Topically, there is some evidence that an external application of green tea may, in some individuals, further irritate an intimate area. Always do a patch test first.

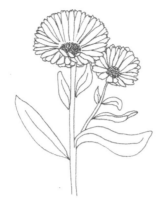

Marigold

Name: Marigold *Calendula officinalis*

    Also known as: Pot marigold, bride of the sun, golds

    Plant family: *Asteraceae* (daisy)

    Part used: Flower heads and petals

    Known constituents: Flavonoids; triterpenes; carotenoids; polysaccharides; phenolic acids; coumarins; essential oil; resins.

    Key words: Sun; warmth; skin healing; female reproductive system.

    Actions: Immune stimulant; anti-inflammatory; anti-fungal; anti-histaminic; styptic; haemostat; diaphoretic; cooling; antibacterial, vulnerary; mildly oestrogenic.

    Emotional uses: Associated with the sun—I always get a real sense of emotional warmth from this beautiful orange-petalled plant. It has been said to comfort the heart and spirit, and to help temper anger, impatience and pent up energy.[31]

    Physical uses: This is one herb I definitely want you to use inside and out! Almost every client that comes to see me will get marigold in their prescription. Fabulous as a gentle anti-fungal, it also helps repair skin injury and tissue damage—useful to know for cuts that need healing elsewhere on the body (use a cream or ointment for this). It's ideal for topical applications in pessaries (I often use a marigold infused oil as a base for pessary making), sitz baths, compresses and gel applications (here I'd also used an infused oil rather than a water extract in a gel). It has also been shown to adhere well to mucous membranes,[33] making it a perfect choice for vaginal health.

I also use it internally orally as a tea or tincture to help with lymphatic clearance of pelvic congestion that may be linked to chronic or recurrent vaginal conditions. It is useful for enlarged lymph nodes—these nodes are an integral part of the immune system, where lymphatic fluid is 'cleaned' by many of the immune components residing in these hot spots of protection and defence. In this application, Marigold is immunomodulatory. I always include it for clients with thrush or cystitis. As a mildly bitter-tasting herb, it's also a liver herb and when taken internally stimulates the flow of bile (all bitter-tasting things have this action, meaning that bitter things are also good for digestion!).

Suggested use: Use both internally as a tea, drinking freely while you clear infection, and externally in sitz baths, compresses and pessaries for thrush. **Combines well with** aloe vera, chamomile, apple cider vinegar externally.

Safety considerations: Considered to be safe at therapeutic levels, with a low risk of allergy.[33]

Sodium bicarbonate (aka bicarbonate of soda)

An alkaline substance that many of us already have in our cupboards, known by the name of baking soda, this is wonderful to use on its own in a sitz bath if cytolytic vaginitis is what's going on for you. The alkaline properties will help to reduce the overgrowth of *Lactobacilli* and will soothe the area. Dissolve 1–2 tablespoons of this crystalline powder in comfortably warm water for each sitz bath and repeat two to three times a week as the *Lactobacilli* dominance is reduced.

Immunity

Marigold

As above. Drink 2–3 cups a day as a tea. Combines well with p'au d'arco, the nervine herbs and the urinary herbs, internally.

Medicinal mushrooms

Not a herb, but rather a fungi; medical herbalists and other professionals working with natural medicine will often recommend medicinal mushrooms because they are considered to enhance the immune response and, indeed, immunity. This is due to their polysaccharide content and type, which are considered to potentiate the immune response.[37] This can be helpful to support the body in all types of vaginal infection. In addition, due to their action on the immune system, they may also be helpful in vaginal conditions where allergy may play an underlying role.

A word of caution here, when sourcing medicinal mushrooms, I strongly recommend against foraging for them yourself as mushroom identification can be tricky and prove deadly if you get it wrong, even with a good guidebook. While you can use a general mix of medicinal mushrooms from a reputable source (see the Resources section for a couple of good options in the UK), making sure they are from an organic source is wise.

The specific species of *Ganoderma lucidum* (reishi), *Lentinula edodes* (Shiitake) and *Pleurotus ostreatus* (oyster mushroom) and *Trametes versicolour* (turkey tail) have been shown to have anti-fungal action against *Candida albicans*,[37] and some components from mushroom cell walls may help to prevent colonisation of the *Candida* species in intestinal muscosa.[37] Because of their immune system modulating effects, they may also be useful in lichen planus and lichen sclerosis.

Dosage: A general dose is 2–3 g a day.

Safety considerations: High-quality mushroom supplements are generally well tolerated, but there are some specifics to take note of: *Ganoderma lucidum*: patients on anti-coagulation medicine should be monitored, although no changes were detected in trials on healthy volunteers.[37] *Lentinula edodes*: some reports of dermatitis from possible raw mushroom consumption, but none reported from those taking supplements.[37] *Pleurotus ostreatus*: caution for raised statin levels in patients taking protease inhibitors such as ritonavir and indinavir, which use some of the same liver enzyme pathways.[37] *Trametes versicolour*: none reported.

Echinacea

Name: Echinacea *Echinacea angustifolia, Echinacea purpurea*

Also known as: Purple cone flower, black sampson

Plant family: *Asteraceae* (daisy)

Part used: Rhizome (root); the whole plant can also be used, although the root is the most widely used in commercial preparations

Known constituents: Phenylpropanoids; alkamides; polysaccharides; trace amounts of essential oil.

Key words: Acute immunity; deep clearing and cleansing.

Actions: Antimicrobial; antiseptic; anti-inflammatory; vasodilator; lymphatic; immune modulation, especially of white blood cell count, T cells and natural killer cells; vulnerary.

Physical uses: Most commonly known for helping reduce the length of a cough or cold, echinacea does a lot more than just that. While studies have shown that if taken in acute doses (5 ml every hour for the first four hours of the onset of a cold or flu), it can shorten the duration of the infection, echinacea can also be used in a variety of other ways. Prior to its modern use for colds, echinacea was used more as an immune system cleanser, helpful for when things had really taken hold in the body, such as deep infections, boils, abscesses, buccal and gastric ulcers, septic wounds, blood poisoning and systemic *Candida*. When used like this, it is taken for longer than for a cold (although many people do take it prophylactically over the winter, it wouldn't be the way I would use it). Studies have shown that echinacea has many pharmacological actions, including immunomodulation, antiviral, antibacterial and anti-fungal activities and that it may be useful in many prescription mixes for a variety of infections.

Suggested use: Echinacea is a good one to add to your tincture mix for almost any vaginal complaint. The modulation action it has on the immune system means that it can be one very useful way to address fungal and bacterial imbalances, supporting the body at the same time.

Dosage: is around 5 ml a day of a commercially available tincture (1:3, 45%).

Combines well with marigold, any of the nervine herbs, any of the digestive herbs and ones specific to what you are experiencing.

Safety considerations: The quality of echinacea available to buy commercially varies. One way to tell if it's of good quality is how tingly it feels on the tongue when you take the tincture. The more tingly it is, the better the quality. If you are taking immunosuppressant drugs or have a progressive systemic disease such as tuberculosis, leukaemia, collagen disorders, MS, autoimmune disorders, AIDS and HIV[30] then its advised to only take echinacea under the supervision of a qualified medical herbalist in case of interaction or unwanted effects. There is a lack of data on the safety of echinacea in pregnancy and lactation,[30] so caution should be exercised.

Vitamin C

Also known as ascorbic acid, vitamin C is a vital co-factor in many metabolic functions and enzymatic reactions. It acts as an antioxidant in the body and contributes to the normal functioning of the immune system. It is a water-soluble vitamin, so any surplus to your body's requirements will be excreted in your urine. It is generally well tolerated, but high doses may cause digestive discomfort, headache, trouble sleeping and flushing of the skin. It is used to prevent and treat scurvy, is essential in wound repair and for the production of certain neurotransmitters.

While I recommend getting vitamin C from good sources in the diet, such as broccoli, kiwi and citrus fruits, berries, rosehips, kale and peppers, if you have a vaginal condition going on I also recommend supplementing up to 1000 mg a day due to its beneficial effect on the immune system and tissue repair. Use good quality supplements that are gentle on the stomach and don't contain fillers or bulking agents— these have just been included to make it convenient to manufacture the tablet or capsule and have no benefit to the body whatsoever; however, they must be processed by the body in order to 'get at' the vitamin or mineral.

Up to 60% of the vitamin C content of food is broken down by heat, so cooking any foods you are eating specifically for their vitamin C content would greatly reduce their vitamin C value. Vitamin C comes in different forms—I recommend ester C to be taken in capsule form for its gentleness on the digestive system. It's handy to have vitamin C in the house, especially if suffering from BV. Using them as pessaries at the onset of a BV infection or during one (described below, p. 159) is a very useful therapeutic tool for this issue in particular. Being of an acidic pH and well tolerated by the body, they can help to bring the vaginal pH back to an acid balance and get the bacteria that cause BV under control.

Vitamin D

Vitamin D is a group of fat-soluble vitamins that have many actions within the body, including assisting with bone health (and preventing rickets, and possibly osteoporosis); immune health (activating the innate immune system and damping down the adaptive immune systems; with overall antibacterial, antiviral and anti-inflammatory effects); possibly reducing symptoms for clinical depression; and normal muscle functioning.

There are five types of vitamin D, but the most important for humans are D_3 (cholecalciferol) and D_2 (ergocalciferol). We mostly obtain these via skin synthesis due to exposure to sunlight and supplementation.

Naturally occurring dietary sources are limited to animal products (D_3) and fungi (D_2), and often processed foods are fortified with it.

As mammals can synthesise vitamin D in their skin via exposure to sunlight, it is technically not actually a vitamin but really a hormone. Produced in this way or taken in from dietary sources, it needs to be activated by two protein enzyme hydroxylation steps in the liver and then the kidneys before it becomes biologically available to us, which can take three to four days. Aside from the immune-enhancing benefits of vitamin D, I also recommend it if you are specifically suffering from aerobic vaginitis or desquamative inflammatory vaginitis (DIV), as deficiency is implicated in the development of this condition.

D_3 may also be useful to supplement with if, on testing, you are deficient in it and are suffering from relapsing UTIs as it may help to stimulate the production of chemical compounds, which play an important role in urinary tract integrity.[54,55] Aside from not eating foods of animal origin, or gaining enough exposure to sunlight, it has been shown that people with dark-coloured skin who live in temperate regions are more likely to be vitamin D deficient due to naturally higher melanin levels than lighter-skinned people, hindering its synthesis. This is explained by melanin working as a natural pigmentation in the skin to protect it from sun exposure. For these people, supplementation may be essential if living in temperate regions.

Dosage: In the UK dosage is recommended at around 10 µg (400 IU) per day, but more may be required depending on starting levels. Choosing a good brand that's easily absorbed, such as BetterYou, ensures you get a good bioavailable form. Although toxicity is rare, and only caused through supplementation, it is something to be mindful of. According to some research, the upper tolerable limit is 100 µg (4000 IU) a day for adults, while others maintain that higher levels sustained over several months may produce toxicity.

Those with hyperparathyroidism may be more sensitive to developing hypercalcaemia in response to an increase in vitamin D. Overdose causes hypercalcaemia which can be evidenced through increased thirst and urination, and if left untreated can cause calcium deposits in the soft tissues and organs such as the kidneys, resulting in organ damage, which may be irreversible. It's best to consult with a qualified healthcare professional before taking vitamin D if you are pregnant or breastfeeding.

Prebiotics

In a world where probiotics are becoming commonplace and their benefits are well known, I'd love to introduce you to their helpful sidekick, prebiotics. Prebiotics act like a food or substrate for the good bacteria that we want to encourage in the gut: *Bifidobacteria* and *Lactobacilli*. Supplementing with probiotics ensures the gastrointestinal environment is well stocked with the food that promotes the growth of any probiotics you go on to take.

Prebiotics are made of non-digestible, soluble fibre such as fructooligosaccharides or inulin, which pass through the bowel without being broken down, and help to promote the elimination of waste via the bowel (which has a benefit in oestrogen dominant conditions such as RVVC and CVVC, see below). I may recommend them when taking probiotics orally; when someone has a particularly poorly balanced gastrointestinal microflora; or as part of a regime for someone with a high oestrogen condition as part of a clearance protocol. Inulin powders are a good way to add prebiotics into your diet, starting with a teaspoonful a day, added to smoothies, juices, porridges, soups or stews. The dose can be then increased or decreased based on your bowel tolerance (it can cause bloating and flatulence in some people until they adjust—if this hasn't improved in 3–4 days, decrease the dose until you are comfortable), until you find a dose that is good for you. Don't use these long term to regulate your bowel movements without seeing a qualified practitioner to ensure you don't become reliant on them.

Probiotic

And so to probiotics, which are said to help with transit time and good bacterial composition, there has been some debate over whether taking probiotics orally can help with vaginal health. And if they can, how does that translocation happen? Bearing in mind that we want the vaginal microflora to be *Lactobacilli*-dominant (not *Bifidobacteria* as you want in the GI tract), it has been shown that probiotics that are taken orally are able to survive the digestive tract and translocate to the vagina and urinary tract.[41] This is wonderful news for women suffering from chronic BV, UTIs and RVVC/CVVC, and probiotics may need to be taken orally over the course of several months to address any dysbiosis here.

Two strains have been extensively trialled and shown to have some efficacy for women suffering from chronic BV, UTIs and RVVC/CVVC if taken orally. These strains are *L. rhamnosus* GR-1® and *L. reuteri* RC-14®[42, 43] and so it would be beneficial to look for a probiotic that contains these strains if you are looking to treat these. For Women blend by Optibac or the Bio.Me™ femme V probiotic by Invivo are two such supplements.

We might also find benefit from probiotics orally if we suspect systemic overgrowth of *Candida* in the gut, which, depending on the strain you take, would help to inhibit the growth of the *Candida*, preventing their colonisation, and producing anti-fungal substances. In recent years it has been popular to suspect systemic *Candida* if you have a RVVC/CVVC; however, it's rare for this to be the case. If you do suspect it, it's worth getting a stool test done privately with a nutritional therapist or medical herbalist to find out before you start treating yourself as though you have.

If you are looking to take probiotics in this way, some other strains to look for are *Saccharomyces boulardii*; *Saccharomyces cerevisiae* CNCM I-3856 (which has been shown to improve the efficacy of conventional anti-fungal treatment,[48] as well as helping to reduce the recurrence VVC, affecting the inflammation process and suppressing *Candida*'s transition from yeast-to-hyphal form); *Lactobacillus acidophilus* NCFM®; *Lactobacillus rhamnosus* GR-1®; and *Lactobacillus reuteri* RC-14®.

Dosage: with oral probiotics dosage would be between 2–6 capsules a day (depending on the severity of the dysbiosis), taken away from meals and hot drinks. The Invivo Bio.Me Femme V are also excellent for using vaginally as a pessary for BV and, with possible benefit, in RVVC/CVVC, as they contain the *L. rhamnosus* strains as well as *L. gasseri* and *L. crispatus*, which are found in predominantly healthy vaginal microbiomes, along with the *L. plantarum* species.

For recurrent BV, use these for seven nights as a pessary following your period, or seven nights in the month if you're post-menopausal, or whenever you have an outbreak. For RVVC/CVVC they can be of use following ovulation if your thrush is cyclical.

Zinc

Zinc is a vital trace element in humans and required for over 300 enzyme functions and 1000 transcription factors. It is the second most abundant trace metal in the human body, after iron, and between 2–4 g of it is distributed through the body, mostly being found in the brain, muscle tissue, bones, kidney and liver, the eye and, in men, the prostate.

Although zinc plays some role in immune health (mild deficiency may impair immunity[40]), and may reduce the severity of the human rhinovirus (common cold) by suppressing nasal inflammation and virus binding and replication at the nasal mucosa, it also is important in a number of major metabolic processes including protein and nucleic acid synthesis.[40] Just a mild deficiency may result in an impaired immune system, as well as an impaired sense of taste, and stunted growth in children.[40]

In the diet, zinc from animal, crustacea and mollusc sources is more readily available than from plant sources, where phytates inhibit absorption. If you choose to supplement in order to support your immunity (and I would only advise this really if you test as deficient) use at least 8 mg daily, to the upper limit of 40 mg daily, and only supplement for the short to medium term.

You should be careful not to overdose on zinc. Signs that you might have are nausea and a bad taste in the mouth. There has been some evidence that people taking 10–33 mg of zinc daily developed copper deficiency, which may indicate that zinc interferes with the utilisation of copper.

Maca

Name: Maca *Lepidium meyenii*
   Also known as: Peruvian ginseng
   Plant family: *Brassicaceae*
   Part used: Root
   I thought long and hard about whether to include maca in this section. In the West in recent years there has been a growing interest in maca as a superfood, purported to increase energy, fertility, libido and overall health. The powdered root can now be bought in supermarkets and from health food shop shelves and I wanted to include it here simply because of its recently increased popularity and reputation. It's not often used in a clinical setting by a Western medical herbalist (but I am sure there are those out there with greater knowledge of traditional Peruvian medicines who may use it), but it is a source of iron and can be helpful in menopause.

In Peru it is often consumed cooked, as part of the diet. It seems that a lot of the actions attributed to it are likely to be because it is a food stuff that is very rich in nutrients and vitamins, so if you are particularly run down it might be helpful to give you some of what you are lacking. Please bear in mind the sustainability and fair trade aspects of this food stuff before reaching for it from the supermarket shelves. If you do decide to try it, you can mix a teaspoon into your smoothie, porridge, or soups per day.

Digestion and elimination

Dandelion

Name: Dandelion *Taraxacum officinalis*
  Also known as: Pissabed, wet-the-bed, lion's tooth, clocks
  Plant family: *Asteraceae* (daisy)
  Part used: Both the leaf and root are used, but have slightly different properties, the leaf being mainly concerned with the kidneys. In this monograph we cover only the root
  Known constituents: Carotenoids; sesquiterpene lactones; vitamins A, B and C; rich in minerals including potassium.
  Key words: Bitter; digestive stimulant; cooling.
  Actions: Cholagogue; bitter; mild laxative; bile duct stimulator; galactagogue.
  Emotional uses: Grounds and strengthens the emotional body, solar plexus and a person's sense of self. Feelings of bitterness and resentment can get 'trapped' in the liver and this liver-stimulating herb can help release those feelings, and 'sweeten' you up.[31]
  Physical uses: Use the bitter-tasting roots to help stimulate digestion and bile release for better waste elimination via the bowels. This is important in vaginal health conditions and in particular RVVC and CVVC, because if oestrogen is dominant in the body due to irregular bowel movements, the extra oestrogen in the system will influence vaginal health. (Irregular bowel movements may mean that 'waste' oestrogen is recirculated by the bowels and liver before getting a chance to be eliminated.)
  Dandelion Root is a mild laxative and bile stimulant, but it can also be used for mild jaundice, lack of appetite and liver disorders.[32] Externally, the milky sap of the fresh root can be applied for warts.
  Suggested use: If you are suffering from a vaginal condition that is affected by higher oestrogen levels, or you are not defecating at least once every day, taking dandelion root internally may be of benefit to you.

Dosage: Take as either a decoction of the roots, 1 cup twice a day, or as a tincture, including 5ml a day of 1:3 45% as part of a mix.

Safety considerations: Do not use if you have occlusion of the bile duct, gallbladder empyema or obstructive ileus.[39] Those with an allergy to the Asteraceae may find they have contact allergy, but you are likely to know if this is you. No allergic reactions have been reported for ingestion.[30]

Cinnamon

Name: Cinnamon *Cinnamonum zeylaniculm*
   Also known as: Blume
   Plant family: *Lauraceae* (laurel)
   Part used: Dried inner bark curls
   Known constituents: Essential oil; polysaccharides; proanthocyanidins; phenolic acids.
   Key words: Warm; sweet; pungent; stimulating.
   Actions: An amphoteric effect on blood sugar levels; carminative; antimicrobial; spasmolytic; anti-inflammatory; anti-nociceptive; appetite stimulant; vulnerary, anthelmintic; circulatory stimulant.[33]
   Physical uses: This lovely warming herb is much beloved of cooking and baking. It can be used therapeutically to help lower blood sugar levels where blood sugar regulation is an issue (although this shouldn't be relied upon as the main means by which it is regulated) and has a long history of being used in this way, dating back to the Still Room recipe books of Tudor England. It can be useful for those who energetically suffer from cold, tired, weak states that may be characterised by lowered immunity. These two qualities alone make it quite a nice choice for vaginal thrush where blood sugar is implicated (it is also worth checking for poorly or un-controlled diabetes in these cases). Cinnamon can also be a useful addition to aid poor, slow digestion especially bloating and spasms, but it only helps symptomatically rather than getting to the cause.
   Suggested use: If you have RVVC that you have noticed is linked to your sugar intake, I recommend reducing dietary sugar and regulating blood glucose as well as ensuring you don't have diabetes by speaking to your GP about taking a fasting glucose blood test. It may help for you to include decent doses of cinnamon in your daily food, such as a teaspoon on your porridge, in a smoothie, or in curries. This will level out peaks and dips in blood sugar, evening out energy, and aid digestion and elimination.

Safety considerations: Contraindicated in pregnancy or possible pregnancy in therapeutic amounts (in foods is ok),[33] and also with stomach and intestinal ulcers.[38] Caution should also be taken for possible allergic hypersensitivity to it, possible toxicity from prolonged use, and a speculative possibility around causing acid reflux.[38]

Chamomile

Name: Chamomile
   Also known as: Mother of the Gut
   Part used: Tea or tincture to settle a griping, irritated, inflamed stomach or digestive tract or to restore regular bowel movements.

Prebiotics — inulin

The use of a FOS type prebiotic fibre can promote healthy and regular bowel movements for improved oestrogen clearance. See the Immunity section above for dosing.

Other ways to improve gut motility

To improve the rate and quality of gut motility with regards to oestrogen clearance and reducing overall stagnation of processes in the pelvic region, there are some other suggestions to consider. These can form part of a healthy lifestyle and are a really good place to start.

Firstly, make sure you are getting enough water intake each day. Although we get water from our food and hot drinks, such as black tea with milk, and coffee, we would be aiming at an additional 2 litres or eight glasses of water a day. When I talk to people about this they often are perplexed as to why we can't include tea and coffee within this water intake allowance. It is because both of these drinks are diuretic, meaning that you urinate out more liquid than you take in—their net effect is essentially one of dehydration. Water is vital for the formation of stools that are easy to pass. If you are even slightly dehydrated, this will impact your bowel movements.

Having adequate exercise during the day is another essential way to ensure regular bowel movements as it encourages peristalsis. Peristalsis is the involuntary muscular movements of the digestive tract, that occurs in progressive wavelike contractions, passing the bolus or food/waste along the system. Have you ever sat on the loo and strained in order to pass your stool? If so, you're not alone. Although in the West we may consider using a lavatory to be the only way to 'go', it actually doesn't work particularly well with the way our bodies are designed. Whether we like it or not, human bodies have evolved to defecate in a squatting position and doing so alleviates much of the pressure on the intestines. While I'm not suggesting changing your toilet habits to such an extreme extent, I am inviting you to try using a small footstool in front of the toilet, to rest your feet on while you go for a number two. It really will take the pressure off your bowel and colon and aids you in passing stools more comfortably.

Abdominal massage, as mentioned above for help with gynae conditions generally and pelvic congestion, can also be helpful to promote digestion and elimination and could be a nice addition to your self-care if constipation is a factor for you. In the first instance, go and see a trained therapist, who will show you how to perform the massage yourself in-between sessions, which is a lovely way to connect with your body as well as helping digestion along.

A note on senna

While the use of the occasional senna product might be helpful if you have an isolated incident of bad constipation, regular use of it can cause the bowel to lose muscular tone, meaning that you need to then rely on it, or other supplements, in order to have a bowel movement. This is because it stimulates your gut to pass stools through irritation, rather than promoting normal function. This is a great example of when natural doesn't automatically mean ideal or without side effects. If you have become reliant on senna or a similar supplement in order to have a bowel movement, I would recommend you work with a qualified health professional to increase your natural function and reduce your reliance on them. Whatever you do, don't just withdraw them and expect the bowels to function as they should.

Mucous membrane integrity

Broadleaf plantain

Name: Broadleaf plantain *Plantago major*
  Also known as: Waybread, common plantain
  Plant family: *Plantaginaceae*

Part used: Leaf

Known constituents: Acids; alkaloids; amino acids, carbohydrates; flavonoids; iridoids; tannins; choline; allantoin; enzymes; fats; saponins; steroids and thioglucoside.[30]

Key words: Cold and dry.[47]

Actions: Anti-histaminic; mucilaginous; diuretic; anti-allergy; lymphatic; anti-haemorrhagic; demulcent; astringent; expectorant; antibacterial.[32]

Physical uses: Wonderful to use fresh and crushed up, externally on bites and stings, this wonderful demulcent has a neuralgic action which is useful when taken internally as a tea as part of a mix for UTIs and haemorrhoids that are bleeding. It's interchangeable with its close relative *Plantago lanceolata* (also known as plantain—the main visual difference being the leaves—round for major, long and pointed for lanceolata). Traditionally used as part of a remedy for thrush, pharmacological studies have shown that one of its constituents, aucubin, has shown antimicrobial activity towards *Staphylococcus aureus*,[32] making it potentially useful in cases of aerobic vaginosis. Its anti-allergy properties means it is of use in RVVC and CVVC where histamines have been shown to play a role in upsetting the vaginal mucous membranes.

Suggested use: If you're suffering from UTIs, use this as one of the ingredients for a urinary tea—up to 17 g a day. If you're suffering from RVVC/CVVC or AV this can be taken orally as part of a tincture mix if you suspect that your condition is being exacerbated by a histamine reaction. Dosage would be around 5 ml a day of a 1:5 tincture. It can also be used topically for the same reason, as a sitz bath. **Combines well with**: Chamomile; Calendula; green tea.

Safety considerations: May cause contact allergy in some individuals so do a patch test first. An excessive dose internally may have a laxative effect and/or have a hypotensive effect.[30]

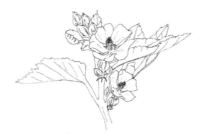

Marshmallow root

Name: Marshmallow root *Althea officinalis*
Plant family: *Malvaceae*
Part used: Root
Known Constituents: Mucilage polysaccharides; flavonoids; phenolic acids; tannins; saponins.
Key words: Cooling; soothing; relaxing.
Actions: Respiratory and urinary demulcent; anti-histaminic; expectorant; emollient; diuretic; anti-lithic; antitussive; vulnerary.[30]
Emotional uses: Has a softening effect.
Physical uses: Wonderful for inflammation of the respiratory tract and the urinary tract, this is a great herb to add into any mix for respiratory, vaginal or urinary infections. The mucilage protects and soothes and seems to have an effect on all mucous membranes in the body, even those it doesn't come into contact with. It is surmised that this is via some sort of reflex action across mucosal membrane sites. As an aside, a poultice or ointment can be made from the powdered root and applied topically for boils, abscesses, ulcers and old wounds, to draw out any waste material.
Suggested use: Use for both UTI and any vaginal conditions where inflammation exists (any vaginitis or VVC) to soothe the mucous membranes. The high mucilage percentage in the root is best extracted as a cold infusion. Mucilage is broken down by heat or by alcohol, so it's not ideal to tincture marshmallow root or to take it as a hot infusion.
Dosage: Use a teaspoon per cup, up to three times a day. The best way to make it is to add the chopped root to a cup of cold water and leave it to stand overnight, covered. Never make more than one day's dose ahead of time and do remember to store it in the fridge.
Safety considerations: None known.[30]

Bayberry

Name: Bayberry *Myrica cerifera*
Also known as: Wax myrtle, candleberry bark, southern bayberry, southern wax myrtle
Plant family: *Myricaceae*
Part used: Root bark

Known constituents: Triterpenes; flavonoids; tannins; starch; resin; a small amount of volatile oils.[33]

Key words: Strengthening the tissues.

Actions: Astringent; mildly diaphoretic; circulatory stimulant; bactericidal; spermatocidal.[33]

Physical uses: Wonderful for conditions that you may think of as wet and loose, such as diarrhoea, mucous colitis, congestive catarrhal conditions of the mucous membranes, vaginal *Candida* and *Leucorrhoea*, this is ideal for vaginal conditions that have copious amounts of discharge. Being so astringent, it also has a traditional use for nasal polyps and various sorts of internal bleeding (I would say practitioner guided use only here), as well as helping to break fevers, and externally for leg ulcers.[32]

Suggested use: Consider using orally as a tincture; topically as a decoction of the root bark as part of a sitz bath mix for any vaginal condition that has a lot of white discharge, but in particular VVC. It may also be useful where an allergy or intolerance is suspected to play a role.

Dosage: Tincture for oral use: not more than 5ml a day. If using as a sitz bath, decoct 1 teaspoon of the root bark in a cupful of water and add to the sitz bath mix when cool.[32]

Safety considerations: Emetic and hypertensive in large doses.[30,33] Not suitable for use in pregnancy, possibility of pregnancy or lactation.[30] Do not take for more than two weeks orally/internally as the tannin content may interfere with iron absorption from food or supplementation.[30]

EFAs

While there are many fats that humans consume through diet, there are only two, known as essential fatty acids (EFAs), that we need to ingest, as we can't synthesise them, but are required for biological processes. They are alpha-linolenic acid (an omega 3 fatty acid) and linoleic acid (an omega 6 fatty acid).

For reference, docosahexaenoic acid (DHA), an omega 3, and gamma-linolenic acid (GLA) an omega 6, which you may also have heard of, are fatty acids too—but are only considered essential for certain conditions or developmental abnormalities. In addition, you may have also heard of omega 9 oils. These are not considered essential, as the body can synthesise them, but they are found in a variety of foods that we consider healthy to consume.

Fatty acids form a large percentage of the lipid molecules utilised by the body and form the three fatty chains that make up triglyceride molecules, along with a glycerol unit.[40] There are three types of triglyceride molecule (saturated, monounsaturated and polyunsaturated) and these are determined by the make-up of the fatty acids used. Our EFAs are polyunsaturated, which are considered one of the 'healthy' types of triglycerides (the saturated triglycerides are considered the bad guys, especially when it comes to cholesterol and cardiovascular health).

EFAs are used by the body to make molecules involved in the inflammatory process, molecules affecting mood and behaviour, and in cell signalling. Fatty acids in general act as building blocks for many other chemicals in the body, including steroid hormones (sex hormones, adrenal hormones), cholesterol (both the good and the bad types), and may be of benefit for dry skin conditions.

They are also implicated in the health and integrity of mucous membranes, and this is why we want to ensure a good supply here, whichever vaginal health condition we are looking at. Maintaining the health of the vaginal mucous membrane will ensure that there is less chance of opportunistic infection via micro-traumas, a good environment for a healthy microbiome to flourish, and will aid natural lubrication.

Although we need all omega fats in the diet (3, 6 and 9) as part of overall health, the typical Western diet is too often heavily loaded with omega 6 sources. The ideal ratio for omega 3 to omega 6 is 1:4 and is often way out! Higher ratios of omega 6 to 3 can promote higher inflammatory states in the body that are implicated in many chronic illnesses such as cardiovascular disease. Omega 6 sources are higher in animal-based foods, while omega 3 is found more readily in plant sources such as nuts, avocados, seeds, and in oily fish. If you eat animals, include plenty of plant-based foods in your diet so that your 3 to 6 ratio doesn't get out of hand. Bringing in omega 9 oils, also from plants, nuts and seeds is also beneficial.

A good animal source of omega 3 oils (EPS and DHA) that is beneficial for vaginal mucosa and that I will often recommend to my patients, is responsibly and cleanly (GOED approved) sourced Cod Liver Oil, which is also rich in vitamins A and D. For vegetarians and vegans, algae sources of EPA and DHA may be used.

If you're taking an omega 3 oil, have 1–3 teaspoons a day during an acute flare-up, bringing it down to 1 teaspoon per day for a maintenance dose, ideally reducing to zero once the likelihood of the condition returning has become minimal.

Sea buckthorn oil

Also rich in fatty acids, in particular omega 7 (but also 3, 6 and 9), and something I often recommend to my patients to improve vaginal mucus membrane integrity, is sea buckthorn oil. Originally found in the Himalayas, but now naturalised around the UK coast, the oil is extracted from the berries. Omega 7 is a key component of mucosal cells and may stimulate skin generation, helping wounds to heal more quickly[45,46] and I recommend taking a teaspoon (or 3 gm if capsules) a day to help improve vaginal mucosa in those suffering from RVVC, CVVC, cytolytic vaginosis, vaginal atrophy and dermatitis.

Nervines and aphrodisiacs

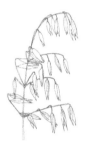

Oats

Name: Oats *Avena sativa*

    Also known as: Oatstraw, milky oat seed

    Plant family: *Gramineae* (grasses)

    Part used: Seeds and tops/straw, rather than oat groats

    Known constituents: Glycosyl flavones; proteins[32]; vitamin E; fixed oil; silicon; manganese; iron; zinc.[49]

    Key words: Nourishing; grounding; nutritive; cooling.

    Actions: Nerve restorative; thymoleptic; mild antidepressant; selective action on the brain and nerve cells; external soothing action on eczema.[32]

    Emotional uses: I have found Oats amazingly useful for emotional grounding and bringing you down to earth.

    Physical uses: Although nerve cells are slow to repair, as they have no direct blood supply of their own to feed them, oats can be very restorative to our nervous system and health if used over considerable time. I prefer to use fresh tincture of milky oat seed, and teas of oatstraw where there is nervous exhaustion, prolonged stress, insomnia and mental irritability. Often vaginal conditions can take a mental, emotional and physical toll on us and can affect our nervous systems (just think of that rich network of nerves serving our pelvic organs and structures). Taking oats either as tincture or oat straw tea can be beneficial to keep us grounded, in our bodies and to help with exhaustion and depletion.

Oats can also be used externally to help with skin conditions and a very traditional way to use them would be with oat groats (porridge oats) tied in the foot of a clean pair of tights and hung over the tap while a bath is being drawn. It can be really soothing for eczema. In a similar way, add oatstraw to a sitz bath to help soothe vaginal and vulval nerve pain.[50] This won't be a one-off treatment so if you are having sitz baths regularly to address pain and inflammation down there, oatstraw will definitely be one of the herbs you want to have in your tool kit.

Suggested use: If you are feeling ungrounded, depleted and generally exhausted by any recurrent or chronic vaginal issue, take fresh milky oat seed tincture up to 5 1/2ml a day, or oatstraw as part of a tea mix, drinking freely. If you are going to add to a sitz bath, include 2–3 handfuls of the oatstraw to each bath.

Safety considerations: None known.

Chamomile

Name: Chamomile

Known constituents: I want to emphasise the emotional component of chamomile, conferring a relaxing and centring feeling of softness, security and nourished wellbeing.[31] I have experienced it bring a feeling of soft roundness to my mood and this can be a useful, if subtle, emotional ally.

Rose

Name: Rose *Rosa* spp.—there are many species of rose that can be used medicinally, including *Rosa Gallica, Rosa damascena, Rosa centifolia, Rosa canina, Rosa rugosa*

  Also known as: Rose
  Plant family: *Rosaceae* (rose)
  Part used: Flower heads, petals and hips (not covered here)
  Known constituents: Tannins; essential oil; vitamin C.
  Key words: Cooling and tonifying.

Actions: Astringent; mild sedative; mild antidepressant; aphrodisiac; increases bile flow.

Emotional uses: Often described as a 'hug in a mug', this gives quite a descriptive idea of how *Rosa* spp. is most often used. Rose can help with self-acceptance, grief, opening your heart, raising the spirits, and indeed is energetically very 'opening'. This is perhaps not the first herb for you if you have emotional trauma that you're not ready to open up to for processing or engaging with, if you don't have very good boundaries with others as it can open you up even further, or if you're in a position where what you are in actual need of is grounding.

Because of its 'opening' energy, it is considered an aphrodisiac. I find it really useful for helping to reconnect to your own sensuality and sexuality—which you can often become disconnected from through shame and discomfort when you have a chronic vaginal health issue. It has a very feminine energy.

Physical uses: The rose family are generally a very 'safe' family of plants, and include not only all the roses, but also fruits such as strawberry, raspberry, blackberry, hawthorn, plum, sloes and apples. Rose is considered to have a tonifying effect on the uterus, as well as increasing bile flow. It's often used in face-care preparations for its astringent effect on the skin,[32] and can be helpful for itching and discharge in VVC, although it wouldn't be my first choice.

Suggested use: It's wonderful to combine the essential oil of rose with that of jasmine (40 drops total of essential oil per 100ml of carrier oil, such as grapeseed or almond) for use as a body oil to help you reconnect to your body and enjoy your sensuality. It can also be drunk as a tea for the same reason.

Dosage: One or two flower heads per cup, allowed to steep, or included as 25 g as part of a tea mix.

Could also be used in a sitz bath mix, adding a handful of dried petals.

Safety considerations: None known.

Ashwagandha

Name: Ashwagandha *Withania somnifera*

Also known as: Indian ginseng, winter cherry

Plant family: *Solanaceae* (potato)

Part used: Many parts of this shrub are used medicinally—we are using the root

Known constituents: Steroidal lactones, including withanolides.

Actions: Adrenally supportive; adaptogenic; sedative.

Physical uses: There's not a great amount of research out there on the lovely ashwagandha. Beloved of Western medical herbalists, it is actually a traditionally used Ayurvedic herb, native to India and known as 'rasayan'; which means 'rejuvenate'. The steroidal components have a similar structure to that of endogenous steroidal components in humans and therefore may have a variety of physiological actions. However, it is mainly used as an adaptogen, which can help the body deal with physiological, mental and chemical stress. It is of particular use for people who are tired, but too wired to sleep well, and is incidentally said to increase egg quality when used over a number of months while trying to conceive. It is included here as many of the patients I see fall within that 'tired and wired' category, often kept awake by their symptoms or a restless brain due to the way we live these days. It's a great herb to use in the background of any mix you decide to make for yourself to support the health of your nervous system and adrenal health.

Suggested use: To support adrenal health if you have been stressed for a while or are having difficulty sleeping.

Dosage: Around 5 ml a day of a 1:5 tincture, as part of a mix.

Safety considerations: Best avoided if you have hyperthyroidism. In addition, there is no data on pregnancy or breastfeeding, so best avoided during this time.

Vitamin B

B vitamins are a series of eight water-soluble vitamins that are required by the body for a variety of physiological processes. Broadly, they support cell health; development of red blood cells; energy levels; eyesight; digestion and appetite; cardiovascular health; muscle tone; and brain and neurological function. Most people can get enough vitamin B from dietary sources, but if you are under stress (and let's face it who isn't in this day and age, let alone dealing with a vaginal health condition on top) or have a condition that affects the absorption of nutrients, you may need to supplement. Signs of actual deficiency are: skin rashes, cracks around the mouth, scaly skin on the lips, swollen tongue, fatigue, weakness, anaemia, confusion, irritability or depression, nausea, abdominal cramping, diarrhoea, constipation and numbness or tingling in the hands or feet. Please note that having one or two of these things doesn't signify that you are deficient in B vitamins, as they are common signs for many different conditions. However, make a sensible assessment and if you are concerned, it's worth booking in with your GP for a test.

Below is a summary of the eight B vitamins:

Thiamin — B₁

Discovered around 1897, thiamin is a co-enzyme used in carbohydrate (and alcohol) metabolism. It has a relatively high turnover in the body and is excreted in the urine. Major deficiency can cause the conditions of beri-beri and Wernicke's encephalopathy, which are rarely witnessed these days. There are no rich food sources of thiamin, but it can be found in wheatgerm and whole wheat products, yeast and yeast extract, pulses, nuts, pork, duck, oats, cod's roe and other meats. The recommended intake per day is 1.0 mg per day for adults. Thiamin has low toxicity.[40]

Riboflavin — B₂

Riboflavin forms part of two oxidising co-enzymes used in intracellular processes, as well as being a co-factor in several enzymes. Deficiency is relatively minor, causing angular stomatitis, cheilosis, atrophy of the tongue papillae, nasolabial dyssebacia and anaemia, or is seen alongside other nutrient deficiencies. Riboflavin is present in most foods, though particularly high sources include milk products, eggs, liver, kidney and yeast. However, riboflavin is unstable in UV wavelength light, and sunlight exposure can greatly reduce the content. The recommended intake per day is around 1.3 mg per day for adults. Riboflavin has low toxicity.[40]

Niacin — B₃

Niacin is the generic term for two compounds that prevent pellagra, which is a deficiency disease characterised by dermatitis, diarrhoea and mental disturbance. Both have equal activity and play a central role in metabolism. Only about half the niacin in the body is from the diet. The other half is synthesised in the liver from tryptophan. Deficiency manifests as pellagra. Food sources include protein-rich foods (tryptophan). Good sources of pre-formed niacin include liver and kidney, other meats, poultry, fish, brewer's yeast and yeast extracts, peanuts, bran, pulses, wholewheat and coffee. Recommended dietary intake works out at about 14 mg for women and 16 mg for men daily.[40]

Pantothenic acid — B_5

Pantothenic acid forms part of co-enzyme A and of acyl carrier proteins which help regulate the disposal of certain breakdown elements of amino acids, as well as lipid synthesis. As pantothenic acid is so widely available in foods, deficiency specifically of pantothenic acid in humans has never been described.

Pyridoxine — B_6

Pyridoxine occurs naturally in three forms that are interchangeable in the body. It forms the major co-enzyme PLP, which is involved in amino acid metabolism, the release of glucose from glycogen stores in the muscles and may also have a role in modulating steroid hormone receptors. Deficiency on its own is rare, but can present as muscle weakness, sleeplessness, peripheral neuropathy, personality changes, dermatitis, glossitis, anaemia and impaired immunity. Pyridoxine is found in a wide range of non- (or lightly) processed foods, including meats, wholegrain products, vegetables, bananas and nuts. Recommended daily intake is about 1.5 mg. Toxicity has been reported in women taking large doses (even doses at 200 mg have been recorded as causing effects) of pyridoxine for PMS or carpel tunnel syndrome, resulting in neuropathy and loss of sensation in the feet.

Biotin — B_7

Biotin is a co-enzyme involved in fatty acid synthesis and catabolism of several amino acids. Biotin deficiency is rare as it's found in a wide range of foods and is produced by intestinal bacteria, but where it occurs it has been associated with red scaly skin rash, glossitis, loss of hair, anorexia, depression and hypercholesterolaemia. The human requirement is estimated to be about 30 µg a day.[40]

Interestingly, there might be a link between biotin and RVVC. It is required by *Candida albicans* for growth and survival, but also by *Saccharomyces cervisiae*, which is a yeast that can competitively inhibit the growth of *Candida* spp. One particular study[52] has shown that one in every 123 individuals is predicted to be a carrier of biotinidase deficiency, and this deficiency has an impact on RVVC. The study showed that supplementing these people with biotin helped to resolve their issues.[52]

Folic acid—B$_9$

Folic acid plays a key role in DNA synthesis, and requirements for it are raised in pregnancy. Deficiency in humans contributes to megaloblastic anaemia—a form of anaemia where red blood cells are enlarged but have a reduced density of chromatin, which is needed for haemoglobin formation. It also affects other blood cell types, and can cause a deficiency of white blood cells. It may also be implicated in infertility and diarrhoea.

In dietary sources of folate, the addition of vitamin C reduces the loss of folate by the heat of cooking, and several drugs, including methotrexate, some chemotherapy drugs and cotrimoxazole may interfere with the metabolism of folic acid. Food sources include green leafy vegetables, liver, kidney, beans, beetroot, bran, peanuts, yeast extract, avocados, bananas, wholemeal bread, eggs and some fish. However, taking a folic acid supplement is twice as bioavailable as folic acid in food stuffs. As an aside, when being treated for pernicious anaemia it is essential to supplement with both folic acid and B$_{12}$, which is covered next.[40]

Cobalamin—B$_{12}$

Coined 'extrinsic factor' in 1948 as a substance found in food that combined with 'intrinsic factor' (something already found in the human gut) that would cure pernicious anaemia, cobalamin is a red compound with the largest molecular weight of all the vitamins. It is involved in a variety of metabolic processes and is infamous for being the B vitamin that vegans may lack as it's most prevalent in animal sources. It's synthesised by micro-organisms and is found in fermented foods or the meat and offal of ruminant animals (as it's created by their gut microflora), shellfish, fish, meat, eggs, milk, cheese and yoghurt. Deficiency is not usually due to the diet, unless vegan, but may be to do with a malabsorption issue in the gut. Overall, B$_{12}$ deficiency causes neurological problems. The recommended daily adult intake is 2.5 µg, and it is difficult to overdose on it.[40]

The majority of people in the Western world, who are living our stressed-out, out-of-sync-with-nature lives, may find it benefits their nervous system to supplement with a good quality spectrum of Bs.

Some great brands include Viridian, Cytoplan, Lamberts and Thorne Research.

Damiana

Name: Damiana *Turnera diffusa*
   Also known as: Curzon
   Plant family: *Passifloraceae*
   Part used: Wild leaves and stems
   Known constituents: Volatile oils; flavonoids; terpenoids; saccharides; phenolics and cyanogenic derivatives.
   Key words: Pelvic bowl activator.
   Actions: Aphrodisiac; nervine; antidepressant; diuretic; stomachic; CNS stimulant; thymoleptic.
   Emotional uses: A wonderful pelvic bowl activator of creative and sexual energy.
   Physical uses: The beautiful herb damiana is one of my favourite herbs for connection to the pelvic bowl, sexual energy and creative awakening. A nervine, and therefore acting on our nervous systems, it is considered an aphrodisiac because of the affinity it specifically shares with the pelvic nerves. Damiana is native to southern Texas, Mexico, South America and the Caribbean, and knowledge of the use of damiana was first recorded and brought to European awareness by the Spanish missionaries that went to try and subjugate South America. They witnessed it being drunk as tea and being smoked as rolled cigarettes, although today in Mexico it has also been used to create a sweet liqueur, that is presented to newlyweds in a voluptuous bottle purported to have been modelled on an Incan goddess!

In the USA in the 1870s, damiana was patented as a medicine that would enhance sexual performance in both men and women. And indeed, the libidinous effects that damiana gives us are felt by all genders. Damiana is a small perennial shrub that grows in semi-arid mountainous regions, and we use its leaves. Most of what we use as medicine is wild-harvested rather than cultivated and should be sourced and drunk with mindfulness, ensuring it's coming from sustainable sources.

Our knowledge of it comes mostly from traditional South American use, and of course our own meetings with the plant, because this is where the (inter)action is! As a nervine it is also an uplifting plant, sightly antidepressant and I have found it to be so from my experiences of being wrapped in its beautiful transcendent nature. As an 'activator' of the pelvic bowl, it has been reported to have a variety of effects on the urinary system; some use it as a diuretic, others for incontinence.

Scientific evidence has been sought to back up damiana's famed reputation as an aphrodisiac, and while this may be not the best way to detect the subtle and complex ways a herb interacts with a person's psychological, emotional and relational sexuality, it has been discovered that some of the constituents isolated from damiana may act in a similar way to steroidal sex hormones, although this cannot explain the aphrodisiac effect.

Suggested use: If you'd like to try this as an aphrodisiac, firstly take it by yourself. Prepare a cup of damiana tea, with a generously heaped teaspoon—steeping, covered, for at least five minutes. When you're ready to drink, pour yourself a cup, noticing the colour of the liquid and deeply inhaling the aroma. Approach it with curiosity. What does it remind you of? Where does it take you? Maybe if journaling here feels right for you, then do, but don't interrupt your flow. When you're ready, imbibe. Take a sip, fill your mouth. How does it make your mouth feel? What images, words, colours are evoked? How does it feel? And how does it feel in your body once you have taken a few mouthfuls? Where can you feel the energy of the plant going and how does it affect your emotions? What comes up and how do you meet it? What movement does it create for you? And what will you do with this energy? How will you use it?

Safety considerations: May interact with iron supplements so leave a gap of several hours between the two.

Siberian ginseng

Name: Siberian ginseng *Eleutherococcus senticosus*
  Also known as: Eleuthero, wild pepper, devil's shrub[30]
  Plant family: *Araliaceae*
  Part used: Root
  Known constituents: Carbohydrates; coumarins; lignin's; phenylpropanoids; triterpenoids; essential oil.[30]
  Key words: Nourishing adaptogen.
  Actions: Anti-stress; adaptogen; aphrodisiac; vasodilator; hypoglycaemic; anti-toxic action; increases immune resistance.[32]
  Physical uses: Not native to the UK, as the name suggests. It has gained popularity here clinically and with the general population as it is

in a class of herbs that can broadly be defined as adaptogens, and indeed this is the main reason I've included it here. Adaptogens are a very useful group of herbs as they help the body 'adapt' to stress. That stress can be defined as chemical stress, psychological stress, physical stress, environmental stress. Research into this class of herbs was first undertaken in Russia in the 1950s as they were looking for herbs that might assist their cosmonauts in their burgeoning space programme. Of course, individual species have their own actions, but as a broad class of herbs, adaptogens can be very useful and share some similarities of action.

I have included this form of ginseng, as opposed to panax or another ginseng, because of its particularly gentle, nourishing activity. It's great for people who are depleted, low on energy reserves and run down. It's not too energetically 'pushy' and I use it a lot to support my patients as an adaptogenic tonic.

Suggested use: Use as a base in a tincture mix for up to a month if you have been suffering a lot of stress, feel depleted or low on energy. It would also be appropriate if you have interrupted sleep. Ultimately, it's very supportive of the nervous system.

Dosage: 5 ml of a 1:5 tincture a day.

Safety considerations: There is the potential for it to interfere with anticoagulant, hypoglycaemic and hypo/hypertensive medicine so it should be avoided in these cases. Also, avoid in pregnancy, suspected pregnancy and lactation. Should not be taken for extensive or long periods of time.[30]

Mimosa

Name: Mimosa *Albizzia julibrissin*
   Also known as: Silk tree, tree of happiness
   Plant family: *Fabaceae* (bean/legume)
   Part used: Flowers and bark
   Known constituents: Saponins; tannins; albitocin; b-sitosterol; amyrin; 3,4, -trihydroxyflavone; spinasterylglucoside; machaerinic acid; lactone; methyl ester; acaci acid; flavinol glycosides and lactone.[53]
   Key words: Happiness.
   Actions: Calming sedative; anxiolytic; antidepressant.[53]
   Emotional uses: Native to China, Persia, Korea and Japan, it is known in the Chinese Materia Medica as a calming spirit herb, where the bark is thought to anchor the spirit and the flowers are thought to lighten it.[53]

It also says that mimosa can be useful for irritability and angry feelings due to constrained emotions that are accompanied by epigastric pain and feelings of pressure in the chest.[53]

Physical uses: I've included it here for its wonderful, uplifting antidepressant and anxiolytic activity, and indeed it is thought to enhance all aspects of neurotransmitter secretion and regulation.[53] Traditionally, it has also been used for the treatment of insomnia, amnesia, sore throat and melancholy.[53]

Suggested use: It's becoming better known that dealing with a recurrent or chronic vaginal health condition can also affect mental health. You may not feel like socialising, need to be near your facilities at home and therefore feel reluctant to go out, are worried you're going to be dealing with it forever and can see no end, feel unattractive and unable to engage in sexual activity ... the list goes on. Albizzia can provide some wonderful light and background support to you while you are on your healing journey (yes, it is a journey, especially as it can take a considerable while to accurately work out and diagnose what is going on for you). After experience with both, I favour working with mimosa over the popular St John's wort for anxiety and depression (St John's, although it has been pigeon-holed in the West as an antidepressant, actually has a broad and rich set of other actions in addition to its antidepressant activity for mild to moderate depression).

Dosage: Around 5 1/2 ml of a 1:3 tincture a day as part of the mix.

Safety considerations: Possible interaction with sedative medicines[53] so please don't take if you are also taking pharmaceutical sedatives.

Jasmine and saffron

I wanted to include a note here on jasmine (*Jasminium officinale*) and saffron (*Crocus sativus*). Neither are often used clinically these days, but both are aphrodisiacs and because of that I wanted to let you know about them.

Saffron is commonly used in culinary delights for its flavour and colour, and anyone acquainted with it can tell you how expensive it is. The stigmata is the part of the plant that is used, with each flower having only three (and a purported 75,000 flowers are needed to make one pound of saffron spice—hence why it attracts the value it does). Containing crocins, volatile oil, fixed oil, pigments, and vitamins B_1 and B_2, it has been traditionally used as an expectorant, diaphoretic and antidepressant as well as an aphrodisiac.[32] Cooking with it could be an interesting way to experiment with aphrodisiacs for yourself and/or with a partner(s).

Another great way to experiment would be with the beautiful jasmine. Traditionally used as a nerve relaxant, astringent and bitter as well as an aphrodisiac, this member of the Olive family contains an alkaloid called jasminine, salicylic acid and resin.[32] A wonderful way to experiment with this plant would be to use the essential oil of jasmine in a body oil (as suggested above in the section on rose), to help you reconnect to your body and enjoy your sensuality.

Hormonal

Fennel

Name: Fennel *Foeniculm vulgare*
  Plant family: *Umbelliferae* (carrot)
  Part used: Seeds
  Known constituents: Essential oil; phenylpropanoids; flavonoids; coumarins; glycosides.
  Key words: Mildly oestrogenic; warming; aromatic.
  Actions: Gently warming digestive; carminative; aromatic; antispasmodic; galactagogue; rubefacient.
  Emotional uses: Fennel is very nourishing and has something of a 'mother' energy about it. It is calm and relaxing and helps to open people up who are in need of emotional nourishment, and who need to learn how to care better for themselves. It is also good for promoting sensuality.[31]
  Physical uses: Well known as 'gripe water' for infant colic, or a nice after-dinner digestive tea, I have included fennel here because of evidence from an Iranian study that showed it was able to help alleviate some of the main symptoms of vaginal atrophy (itching, bringing, dryness and dyspareunia) in post-menopausal women, as well as improving the pH and cell health of the vagina in these circumstances.[44] This is very helpful for women who would prefer to use natural methods rather than HRT to improve the situation.
  Suggested use: Use an infused fennel oil to make a cream or pessary and apply high in the vagina as often as needed if you are suffering from mild vaginal atrophy or BV related to low oestrogenic conditions.

Dosage: For digestive issues such as bloating, you can take a teaspoon of fennel seeds per cup of tea, infusing for five minutes, up to three times a day.

Safety considerations: Used vaginally, please avoid in pregnancy. I wouldn't expect there to be further safety considerations as long as you are ensuring anything you are making and applying is done in a very hygienic way, and you don't have a known allergy to fennel.

Red clover

Name: Red clover *Trifolium pratense*
  Also known as: Beebread, trefoil
  Plant family: *Fabaceae* (bean/legume)
  Part used: Flowers
  Known constituents: Glycosides; coumarins; flavonoids; isoflavones including daidzein, biochanin A and genistein; saponins; resins; minerals; vitamins.[32]
  Key words: Hot and dry.
  Actions: Alterative; phyto-oestrogenic; de-obstructant; anti-spasmodic; sedative; expectorant;[32] mildly astringent.[30]
  Emotional uses: Useful for those who hold onto strong, negative emotions and seem unable to let them go, such as grief, depression, sorrow, worrying and over-thinking.[31]
  Physical uses: As a deep-acting blood cleanser it can be useful for skin conditions such as eczema and psoriasis, as well as mouth ulcers and gout, and can be useful for conditions where overgrowths are a feature. It is also relaxing for the nervous system and can be used for anxiety and headaches, although this wouldn't be its primary action for us here. Utilising red clover for its oestrogenic properties, conferred by its isoflavone content, may serve anyone experiencing vaginal conditions resulting from lowered oestrogen levels, such as BV postmenopause or vaginal atrophy.
  Suggested use: Where you know without question (by a hormone level blood test or if you are post-menopausal, for example, rather than supposition) that low oestrogen is part of the picture of your vaginal health condition, consider adding red clover into your tincture mix to see if it makes an impact. Only use if oestrogenic foods (see below) do not make a significant difference in the first instance.
  Dosage: 4 ml a day of a 1:10 tincture.[30]

Safety considerations: Not for long-term use without professional advice. Due to the oestrogenic isoflavones, avoid during pregnancy, possible pregnancy and lactation. Caution and professional advice are needed in hormonally-dependent breast cancer, or for anyone taking hormonal medication such as HRT.

Phyto-oestrogenic foods

Phyto-oestrogenic foods are foods that contain compounds that are similar to our own oestrogens but exert a much weaker effect. They work by binding to our oestrogen receptor sites. If we have low levels of endogenous oestrogen, such as in the menopause, they can give us a small oestrogenic-type benefit that may improve our vaginal health, if it's making you prone to BV or you are suffering from vaginal atrophy. In conditions where oestrogen is in excess, they can actually reduce the effects of our own circulating oestrogens by competitively binding with some of our oestrogen receptors.

Below are some foods which contain phytoestrogens (isoflavones and lignans)—try and add some of these into your daily diet where you can.

- Soybeans, sprouted soybeans or soy germ—not soy mince or flakes
- Miso and tempeh
- Alfalfa or sprouted alfalfa—great in salads
- Red clover sprouts—likewise great in salads
- Lentils
- Kidney beans
- Linseeds—not the oil—these need to be pre-soaked before eating, but can then be used in soups, and porridge or cereal.

pH modulation

pH test strips

pH test strips can be a wonderful diagnostic tool alongside your symptoms to help you work out what you have going on (always get microscopy and culture from your GP if you are not clear). As we already know, BV-causing bacteria like to live in a more alkaline environment than the vagina normally provides in health. In a healthy state, the vagina's pH is quite acidic at around 3.8–4.5. A reading heading towards 5 or higher means we may need to consider if these microbes are part of the cause of your symptoms. VVC seems quite happy in the relative acidity of the normal vaginal range and so, if the results still fall within this range, you can consider candidiasis as a possible diagnosis.

To take readings, buy some strips that graduate in 0.1 pH sensitivity. These can be picked up quite easily on the internet and can often be found on websites concerned with water testing. To take a sample to test, use a clean unused cotton bud to catch some vaginal discharge and then place it on the test strip, waiting for up to a minute for any changes in colour to occur. The best time to take the test is when your symptoms are at their worst. You can take it at daily or weekly intervals to indicate how your body is responding to treatment.

Probiotics as pessaries

To aid the restoration of the vaginal microbiome in the case of BV, AV, Mollicutes, UTIs, and to help ensure the dominance of the *Lactobacilli* species, the probiotics that you are taking orally can also be used vaginally as a pessary you use overnight. Although less 'messy' than other pessaries, I would still advise wearing a pad or towel overnight and for the first part of the morning as using probiotics like this can cause a very slight, watery discharge.

Use for seven nights following your period or when you start to experience symptoms, and I really recommend this method for helping to create a healthy dominant population of *Lactobacilli*, rather than using antimicrobial agents directly on the area, which can strip good as well as bad microbial colonies. See the resources section (p. 190) for good brands to use.

Apple cider vinegar (ACV)

This is a rich vinegar made from apple cider that is further fermented to turn the alcohol into acetic acid. Using an organic ACV ensures that it contains what is known as 'the mother', containing enzymes, proteins and, most importantly to us, beneficial bacteria. This, combined with its acidity, makes it a perfect candidate for adding to sitz baths for any condition that raises the pH of the vagina, such as BV. It also has anti-fungal properties, which makes it useful as part of a protocol for VVC.

Dosage: Use 1–2 cups per sitz bath.

Sodium bicarbonate (aka bicarbonate of soda)—as above (pg. 124).

Antimicrobial

Barberry

Name: Barberry *Berberis vulgaris*
    Also known as: Jaundice berry, pepperidge, sowberry
    Plant family: *Berberidaceae*
    Part used: Root bark
    Known constituents: Isoquinoline alkaloids in berberine; tannins; resins polysaccharides and chelidonic acid.
    Key words: Antimicrobial.
    Actions: Antimicrobial; liver stimulant, cholagogue; alterative; uterine stimulant; anti-inflammatory; antiemetic; digestive; febrifuge; anti-diarrhoeal.
    Physical uses: I've included barberry because of its well-known antibacterial activity, which is helpful in vaginal infections such as BV, AV and mollicutes. Extract of barberry bark has demonstrated activity against both gram-positive and gram-negative bacteria,[33] and the inhibition of bacterial adherence to mucosa, which may explain its anti-infection activity.[33] It has also been shown to have anti-inflammatory activity as well as enhancing uterine contractions.[33]

Traditionally, it has been used for liver disorders, including gallstones, cholecystitis and jaundice that has no obstruction of the bile ducts, protozoal infections, eczema, psoriasis, eye infections[33] and leucorrhea.[32]

    Suggested use: Consider using internally as part of a tincture mix in cases of BV, AV and Mollicutes, as well as stubborn cases of RVVC or CVVC where there might be mixed infection and inflammation.[33]

    Dosage: Around 7 ml a day of a commercially available tincture (1:5, 60%).

    Safety considerations: Do not use if you are pregnant or think you might be; have bile duct obstruction because of gallstones, cholangitis, bile duct cancer or pancreatic cancer; any liver or kidney disease; if you suffer from intestinal spasm; or if you suffer from septic gall bladder inflammation. It may also potentiate a range of medication so seek professional advice if you are taking anything pharmaceutical.[38]

Old man's beard

Name: Old man's beard *Usnea* spp.

Plant family: *Parmeliaceae*

Part used: Branch-like lichen growth

Known constituents: Lichen acids including usnaric, thamnolic and usnic acids; vitamin C; possible polysaccharides, mucilage, anthroquinones, fatty acids and carotene.[56]

Key words: Cooling and bitter.

Actions: Antibiotic; expectorant; anti-fungal.

Physical uses: Old man's beard is a lichen. Lichens are not strictly plants, but rather a symbiotic entity created by a relationship between a fungal base and an algae which grows atop, providing food sugars for both parties, made by collecting and converting sunlight! Old man's beard is so-called because it appears as grey-green hair growing from pines, oaks, Douglas fir, apple trees and other fruit trees growing in the Northern Hemisphere.[56] The *Usnea* species are the most common source of the antibiotic and anti-fungal lichen acids and are collected together here as one entry as they are interchangeable for our purposes.

Traditionally used for conditions of the mucous membranes,[56] the lichen acids have been found to be effective against gram-positive bacteria such as *Streptococcus* and *Staphylococcus* that might be implicated in aerobic vaginitis (but not gram-negative enteric bacteria such as *E. coli*).[56] It appears not to affect gastric bacteria as pharmaceutical antibiotics might. It is thought that usnic acid works by disrupting the cellular metabolism of the gram-positive bacteria.[56] It is also clinically useful as an anti-fungal.[56]

Suggested use: Best used as a tincture (you may need to see a herbalist to source this), as the usnic acid is poorly soluble in water, and much better extracted in alcohol. It is best to start with a lower dose and increase if well tolerated by the gut. Fabulous to include with bacterial and fungal vaginal conditions, especially as it has an affinity with the mucous membranes.

Dosage: Start with a dose of around 3 ml a day, rising to the maximum of 4 ml a day if well tolerated.

Safety considerations: Only use the tincture if diluted as it can be irritating for the digestive tract. Always source from a trusted practitioner supply. Avoid in pregnancy, possibility of pregnancy or lactation.

Garlic

Name: Garlic *Allium sativa*
  Also known as: Ajo, allium
  Plant family: *Alliaceae* (onion)
  Part used: Bulb
  Known constituents: Enzymes including alliinase; sulphur-containing volatile oils in alliin and allicin; proteins; amino acids; lipids; prostaglandins;[30] B vitamins; minerals.[32]
  Key words: Warming and bitter.
  Actions: Bacteriostatic; anti-parasitic; antiviral; antiseptic; fungicide; diaphoretic; hypoglycaemic; cholesterol-lowering; expectorant; anthelmintic; anti-histaminic; anticoagulant; antibiotic.[32]
  Physical uses: Recognised in many traditional medicinal systems as being of value, garlic is of great use in many infectious situations such as those affecting the respiratory system and ear canal, and in *Candida* and parasitic infection. Garlic has a plethora of other uses, such as lowering total cholesterol, raising HDL cholesterol levels, lowering blood pressure and anticoagulant activity, among many others. We want to harness its powers here for its antimicrobial activity. When preparing garlic, it is important to crush it as this breaks down the cell walls allowing alliinase and alliin to come into contact with each other, which activates the other therapeutically active sulphur-containing constituents.[30]
  Suggested use: I see recommendations all over the internet for the use of a garlic clove intra-vaginally for thrush. I wouldn't recommend doing this without practitioner supervision and direction, particularly because there can be issues of removal, it can really burn, and also because of its strongly antibiotic properties, which can strip out the good bacteria from the vaginal environment.

Instead, for vaginal conditions, I would consider adding one clove daily into your diet in the first instance. I often talk about adding raw, crushed garlic to dishes, just before you serve, mixed into rice dishes, salad dressings or in sandwiches. This is easy to do as you're probably already accustomed to having it cooked in food. Avoid eating raw on its own as this will undoubtedly cause gastrointestinal discomfort. The next best way I would use it may be in oil-based pessaries, where a garlic-infused oil is used, along with other excipient ingredients.

Safety considerations: As above. If you are about to undergo surgery, it is advised to stop taking garlic therapeutically for two weeks before as it thins the blood. Likewise, do not ingest at this therapeutic level if you are taking anticoagulant or anti-platelet medicines, and seek advice from a qualified practitioner if you are taking other medicines. Avoid in pregnancy, possibility of pregnancy or lactation.[30]

Thyme

Name: Thyme *Thymus vulgaris*

Plant family: *Lamiaceae* (mint)

Part used: Leaves and flowering tops

Known constituents: Volatile oils in thymol and carvacrol; flavonoids; caffein acid; oleanolic acid; ursolic acid; rosmarinic acid; resins; saponins and tannins.

Key words: Aromatic; hot and dry.[31]

Actions: Carminative; anti-spasmodic; anti-tussive; expectorant; antibacterial; anthelmintic; astringent;[30] antiviral; anti-fungal.

Emotional uses: Having the quality of soaring high like the eagle, Thyme can be helpful if you feel that you've hit rock bottom.[31]

Physical uses: Beloved of those experiencing colds, sore throats, mouth ulcers and coughs, this is one herb that you can easily grow in your outdoor space that will have a multitude of uses, including culinary. It is often added to Mediterranean dishes, not only for its taste but also for its digestive benefits. I've added it here for its antimicrobial and anti-fungal activity. It has an affinity for the mucous membranes and may have activity against *Streptococcal* infection.

Suggested use: Can be added to a tea or tincture in both BV, AV and RVVC.

Dosage: If using as a tincture dose at 5 1/2 ml a day of a 1:5 tincture. If using as a tea, you can put as much as 11 g a day into a mix. I would recommend using this as an adjunct support rather than a primary choice in your remedy.

Safety considerations: I would advise against using this in any topical application as the volatile oil may irritate mucous membranes. Do not take Thyme essential oil internally. If pregnant, possibly pregnant, breastfeeding or taking other medication, please take under advice from a qualified health professional.[30]

Vitamin C

A randomised, double-blind, placebo-controlled, parallel-group clinical trial in 2013 showed that using capsules of 250 mg of vitamin C (ascorbic acid) powder as pessaries for six nights a month for six months, following treatment by traditional antibiotics, halves the risk of recurrence for bacterial vaginosis.[57] This is a big deal and a very useful tool to have in your medicine cabinet at home if BV is something you get often. The acidic vitamin C helps maintain and modulate the pH environment that the useful *Lactobacilli* colonies love so much and we want to encourage.

They can be used as pessaries prophylactically or as part of your overall treatment for recurrent BV (if you are using it this way, use it for the first six nights following your bleed or, if you are post-menopausal, for six consecutive nights of your own choosing per month). Insert as per the instructions for using a pessary above—you may find it easier to wet the capsule first with some fresh water to aid insertion. This is particularly helpful if you are post-menopausal. Again, wear a pad overnight and first thing the following morning as it is normal to have a powdery discharge, a warm sensation and gush of wet fluid as part of using the capsule in this way. It's best to avoid intercourse while using.

Lactic acid gel

Lactic acid gels are available over the counter without prescription in the UK and have been shown to be effective at helping treat mild cases of BV and early-stage recurrence of it,[58] and can be used preventatively. It also has the added benefits of fewer side effects than traditional GP-prescribed antibiotics—in studies women much preferred using it because of easy application, once a day.[58]

The rationale behind the use of lactic acid gel is that it helps to re-establish *Lactobacilli* dominance, through re-acidification of the vaginal environment, and wrests away control from the overgrowth of BV-causing microbes. One study showed that 88% of women treated with lactic acid gel for BV showed no signs of BV recurrence, compared to 10% of the placebo group, and that 83% then went on to re-establish a *Lactobacilli*-dominant vaginal ecology.[59]

If recurrent BV is going on for you, try using the gel for seven consecutive days, then apply prophylactically for three days a month for six months. It is best not to mix lactic acid gel with vitamin C at the same time. Try one for the full treatment length (6–7 days) and then leave a good gap of several days to a week in-between if you would like to try the other approach.

Probiotics as pessaries

Similarly, as lactic acid gel may prove useful to help establish a favourable *Lactobacilli* environment, the use of probiotics as vaginal pessaries, as explained above, can also be a way to achieve this. Useful to control the overgrowth of BV-causing microbes, AV, Mollicutes and UTIs, it might also be helpful in situations of RVVC. Use as described above.

N-acetyl-cystine

N-acetyl-cystine or NAC for short is the stabilised form and precursor to the amino acid L-cystine. It has been used as a supplement since the 1960s, when it was found to have mucolytic and biofilm busting properties useful for patients with cystic fibrosis.[60] Since then, it has been found to have many functions in the body, such as the inhibition of certain inflammation pathways, among many others. It has been found to decrease the viscosity of mucous by reducing the size of mucoprotein molecules, and, very importantly, has been shown to be a promising adjunct therapy to use alongside antibiotics (if that's the route you decide to go down) against bacterial biofilms that might exist in dealing with stubborn cases of BV. One systematic review paper[61] reports that not only does NAC reduce the variety of bacteria in a biofilm, but it may reduce the extracellular production of the polysaccharide matrix of the bacteria, while promoting the disruption of the formed biofilm. This is exciting stuff because so often the antibiotics that are prescribed for BV don't really get to the heart of the problem as they tend to be ineffective for biofilms. The answer lies in breaking down that biofilm!

It should be said that if you do take antibiotics (and in some cases you might want to) it's worth rebuilding your gut and vaginal microbiomes again afterwards with the appropriate pre- and probiotics.

If you decide to use NAC for biofilm build-up and resistance in BV, it's best to do so under the guidance of a qualified health professional. They should not be taken if you are on nitrate vasodilators and related medication as it may increase the risk of hypotension. You may need to build-up the dose slowly to a tolerable therapeutic level as sensitive individuals may find it initially causes gastrointestinal upset, headaches, skin rashes, or muscle/joint pain, and for these reasons professional help should be sought. However, this is still an important inclusion in your therapeutic arsenal if you suffer from stubborn BV.

Sodium bicarbonate (aka bicarbonate of soda)

Very useful for controlling populations of *Lactobacilli* overgrowth in cytolytic vaginosis, used as above.

Anti-fungal

Aloe vera

As above. I wouldn't rely on this to be a first-line anti-fungal, but the gel is a great carrier for adding other things too!

Marigold

As above. I want to emphasise what a wonderful and gentle anti-fungal this is. Use it as the backbone of any remedy for VVC.

Garlic

As above.

Thyme

As above.

P'au d'arco

Name: P'au d'arco *Tabebuia impeteginosia*
   Also known as: Lapacho tree, taheebo, ipe roxo, pink trumpet tree
   Plant family: *Bignoniaceae*
   Part used: Inner bark—cambium layer
   Known constituents: Lapachol;[38] Laprachol.[32]
   Key words: Warming.
   Actions: Aids immune system health; antimicrobial; analgesic; anodyne; diuretic; anti-fungal; anti-*Candida*; febrifuge;[32] anticoagulant;[38] aphrodisiac![62]
   Emotional uses: My personal experience with this herb has been very comforting. It has a delicious smoky flavour if drunk as a tea and is very grounding and solidifying.

Physical uses: Used as a medicine by the Inca people for over 1000 years, p'au d'arco has a multitude of uses and a reputation as a great herb to support cancer patients. It is also traditionally used for diarrhoea, boils, leprosy, fever, pharyngitis, snakebite and wounds.[32] However, we will be using p'au d'arco for its anti-fungal and specifically anti-*Candida* effects. Not only is it helpful in the management of VVC, but it can also be a supportive treatment for oral candidiasis too.

Suggested use: The easiest way to bring p'au d'arco into your regime for VVC is via tea. Always ensure you are sourcing your p'au d'arco from a sustainable source, such as Rio Health, as the tree is a giant hardwood, native to the Amazon rainforest.

Dosage: Take 3–4 cups a day using a fresh tea bag each time. You could also add a teabag to a soothing sitz bath.

Safety considerations: There is some question as to whether the Lapachol constituent in P'au d'arco might be an abortifacient and so it is best to avoid in pregnancy or possible pregnancy. Also, avoid if taking anticoagulant medication such as warfarin, as this may potentiate its effects. Seek advice if you are taking any immunosuppressant medication.[38]

Olive

Name: Olive *Olea europea*
Plant family: *Oleaceae*
Part used: Leaves
Key words: Bitter and astringent.[49]
Actions: Hypoglycaemic, antiviral; antibiotic; anti-fungal and anti-parasitic.[49]
Physical and suggested uses: Use of olive leaf fell out of fashion for a while and has only recently made a minor come back. I've added it because it's one that you might consider using for its anti-fungal properties. There are mixed reports about what it is able to inhibit and because of that, along with personal experience, I would only use it as a supportive adjunct, as a tea or in a sitz bath. It can also be used as a supportive remedy in UTIs. It is also worth mentioning here that olive leaf bach flower remedy may be useful to take if you feel exhausted, or have low energy, either in general or because of any vaginal condition.

Dosage: Take three drops under the tongue morning and evening until you feel the situation improving.

Safety considerations: None known, but if you have low blood pressure, please seek advice before taking internally.

Oregano

Name: Oregano *Origanum vulgare*
  Also known as: Wild oregano
  Plant family: *Lamiaceae* (mint)
  Part used: Leaves and flowering tops
  Known constituents: Flavonoids; triterpenoids; vitamins A & C; volatile oil.[49]
  Key words: Pungent and warm.
  Uses: Traditionally used for tinnitus, respiratory tract infections, digestion and *Candida*,[49] I've included this here because oregano oil capsules are popularly seen in health stores and often taken orally for yeast overgrowth. Some people find them very useful, but we don't use oregano in this way in the practice of traditional Western herbal medicine and I would like to encourage you not to either. This is because, while oregano may be a good antimicrobial, taking it in this way concentrates the volatile oils, which would effectively strip out the microbiome. The approach to use here is to rather build a robust microbiome using other methods, not strip out what is already there. In addition, I actively advise against using oregano oil capsules intra-vaginally.
  Dosage: If you would like to work with this herb for its anti-fungal properties, take it as a tea (not a sitz bath), using a pinch of the dried or fresh leaves per cup and steeping for five minutes, up to 3 cups per day, or in food.
  Safety considerations: Avoid in pregnancy, possible pregnancy and lactation.[38]

Caprylic acid

Also known as octanoic acid, caprylic acid is a medium-chain, saturated fatty acid and a carboxylic acid often used as a supplement. It is found in coconut oil, palm oil and the milk of many mammals (including humans) and bovines (cows). Most often extracted from coconut oil in supplement form, it exhibits anti-fungal, antibacterial and anti-inflammatory properties and can also affect cholesterol levels. Effective for those suffering from VVC, it is thought it may break down the membrane of *Candida* cells, as well as arresting yeast-to-hyphal transition.[63] Dosage is around 150–300 mg a day in capsule form, orally, and it is generally well tolerated. Avoiding if pregnant, possibly pregnant or breastfeeding.

Urinary

Olive leaf—as above.

Bearberry

Name: Bearberry *Arctostaphylos Uva ursi*
   Also known as: Kinnikinnick, spreng
   Plant family: *Ericaceae*
   Part used: Dried leaves
   Known constituents: Hydroquinones; iridoids; tannins; phenolic acids; triterpenes.[39]
   Key words: Hot and dry;[31] mild urinary-septic.
   Actions: Diuretic; urinary antiseptic; astringent; styptic; oxytocic,[32] anti-inflammatory.[30]
   Emotional uses: Associated with the base chakra or energy centre, it can help with feelings of victimhood, fear and violent aggressiveness, helping you find courage and your own power without needing to try to exert power over others.[31]
   Physical uses: A key herb for cystitis, painful urination and interstitial cystitis, traditionally it was also used for chronic leucorrhoea,[32] which was considered to be non-specific copious white vaginal discharge (*hint, it's never non-specific and with today's testing technology it's possible to find out what is going on!). It has been found to have activity against *Staphylococcus aureus, Bacillus subtilis, E. Coli, Mycobacterium smegmatis, Shigella sonnet* and *Shigella flexneri*.[30] Clinical studies have shown that bearberry's astringent action is specific to the urinary mucous membrane lining the urethra.[30] There are several constituents that are thought to contribute to the antibacterial activity, and one study posits that one of those constituents even utilises the activity of the pathogenic bacteria which is causing the infection, although none of these constituents have ever been found in the urine.[39] What is clear is that bearberry acts upon the urinary microbiome.
   Suggested use: If you are wanting to treat a 'water' infection, how better to do it than with a water preparation of herbs, a tea! A tea helps

to flush the whole urinary system through and is ideal. Always use bearberry as part of a tea mix.

Dosage: Around 4 g a day in a tea mix, and I would augment any tea treatment plan with probiotics used vaginally as pessaries to target the urinary microbiome.

Safety considerations: Do not use in pregnancy, possible pregnancy or lactation, nor in kidney disorders. Large doses can induce nausea and vomiting. Do not use it for more than two weeks without consulting a practitioner.[32] Take away from food, due to the tannin content.[30]

Cornsilk

Name: Cornsilk *Zea mays*

    Also known as: Maize silk, stigmata maidis

    Plant family: *Gramineae* (grasses)

    Part used: Dried stigma and style

    Known constituents: Amines; fixed oils; saponins; tannins; allantoin; bitter glycosides; flavone; gum; phytosterols; pigments; resin, vitamins C and K.[30]

    Key words: Urinary irritation.

    Actions: Antilithic; mild stimulant; urinary demulcent; diuretic.[32]

    Physical uses: You've probably come into contact with cornsilk when you've cooked a corn on the cob. Those stringy strands that can get stuck in your teeth if you haven't carefully removed them all alongside the green leaves which encase each cob are the very stuff of this entry. Traditionally used as a dried herb for cystitis, overactive bladder, urinary retention, pus in the urine, and urethritis, it is a wonderful addition to any tea for a UTI or feeling of urinary urgency that can often accompany cystitis or a vaginal infection as it's so soothing to the urinary mucous membranes (unless allergic). Hardly any clinical studies have been undertaken on this herb—much of its use relates to empirical use and experience.

    Suggested use: As with most of the urinary herbs taken for the express purpose of dealing with a UTI or urinary irritation, Cornsilk is best taken as a tea and blends well with buchu and bearberry.

    Dosage: Around 14 g a day of the dried herb as part of a blend.

    Safety considerations: Possible interaction noted for therapeutic doses for pregnancy so avoid at this level in pregnancy, possible pregnancy and lactation.[30] Also, avoid if a known allergy.

Buchu

Name: Buchu *Agathosma betulina*
   Also known as: *Barosma betulina*, bucco
   Plant family: *Rutaceae*
   Part used: Leaf
   Known constituents: Flavonoids; volatile oils; resin;[30] mucilage.[32]
   Key words: Urinary antiseptic.
   Actions: Stimulant diuretic and specifically promotes secretion of urine; urinary antibacterial; urinary tract anti-inflammatory.[32]
   Physical uses: Another urinary herb that is under-studied, buchu is traditionally used as an effective urinary antibacterial and anti-inflammatory, and for cystitis, urethritis, prostatitis and acute catarrhal cystitis.[30]
   Suggested use: I always use a combination of buchu, urva ursi and cornsilk whenever I am seeing a patient with a urinary issue. They work well together, and then I add in any other herbs that would also support the person in front of me. And yes, you've guessed it, I use them in a tea! Buchu has a wonderful flavour and has been likened to blackcurrant. I could enjoy it on its own as a pleasant-flavoured beverage (although I'd have to watch the diuretic qualities and cautions below).
   Dosage: Again up to 14 g of the dried herb a day in a tea mix.
   Safety considerations: Buchu should not be taken in higher doses than recommended as it contains a volatile oil that may, in large doses, have the potential to cause toxicity to the liver. With this in mind, avoid in pregnancy, possible pregnancy and lactation.[30]

Nettle

Name: Nettle *Utica dioica*
   Also known as: Stinging nettle
   Plant family: *Urticaceae*
   Part used: Leaves; the roots and seeds are also used in herbal medicine
   Known constituents: Chlorophyll; vitamins including C; acetylcholine; histamine; serotonin; flavonoids glycosides; minerals including calcium, potassium and silicon; lignans.[30, 32]
   Key words: Mineral-rich and anti-histaminic.
   Actions: Diuretic; eliminates uric acid from the body; anti-histaminic; re-mineraliser; antiseptic; styptic; anti-inflammatory; anti-rheumatic; hypoglycaemic; hypotensive; vasodilator; galactagogue; astringent.[32]

Emotional uses: Nettle is a herb for building you up physically and emotionally, and has a fiery element to it. It can help to shift water-logged emotions and emotional 'stuckness'.[31]

Physical uses: The whole Nettle plant, including the roots and seeds, is associated with the urinary tract and its associated structures. Here we look at the diuretic leaf, fabulous for pushing herbal medicine where we want it to go. Rich in minerals, it has a traditional use of 'building someone up' after a long illness and for failure to thrive in children. Nettles have also been used for eczema and rheumatic conditions, and because of their tannin content and galactagogic action there is a history of use for uterine haemorrhage, following childbirth.[30]

Suggested use: Add into a mix where there is a known histamine intolerance in both urinary issues and vaginal ones. Many foods contain histamine, and if this is contributing to your issue you can be advised to try to eliminate them from your diet. Alongside this, I would add in an anti-histaminic herb such as Nettle or Marshmallow. If your issues are more urinary, I would pick Nettle (Marshmallow for more vagina related issues). It's a lovely building diuretic, and again, yup, I'm recommending it as a tea!

Dosage: Dried herb is around 10g daily, spread over up to 3 cups daily.

Safety considerations: Avoid in pregnancy, possible pregnancy and lactation.[30]

Cranberry

Name: Cranberry *Vaccinium macrocarpon*

   Also known as: Mossberry

   Plant family: *Ericaceae*

   Part used: Juiced berries

   Known constituents: Citric acid; malic acid; quinic acid; benzoic acid; fructose; oligosaccharides; anthocyanin; proanthrocyanidins;[30] D-mannose.

   Key words: Urinary antibacterial.

   Actions: Urinary antibacterial; antiscorbutic (anti-scurvy).[32]

   Physical uses: The pharmacological antibacterial activity of cranberry was thought to be due to the fact that it worked to acidify the urine, thereby inhibiting bacterial growth. However, it has been shown that it also inhibits bacterial adherence to the urinary mucosal surfaces, which is an important step in halting the development of a UTI. In practice, there is limited data in clinical studies to prove that cranberry makes a significant difference, although empirical experience may differ.[30]

Suggested use: Some consider it an old wives' tale to use cranberry juice at the first sign of a UTI, but it can be helpful as an adjunct to the main treatment only if you use a juice that has no added sugar. The addition of sugar, although making the cranberry less sour and more palatable, changes the pH, as well as potentially increasing the food source for the offending bacteria. If deciding to add cranberry juice into your therapeutic plan, note it will prove most effective at the first signs of a UTI. It would be best not to rely on this alone to resolve the issue. Only use a sugar-free juice, and drink freely, noting the warning below.

Safety considerations: There have been reports of cranberry interacting with warfarin and affecting international normalised ratios (INRs), or how long it takes your blood to clot, so if you are on this medication then you should avoid cranberry.[30]

D-mannose

A type of sugar with a chemical structure similar to that of glucose, D-mannose is usually available as capsules or powders that can be dissolved and taken in water. It occurs naturally in cranberries, apples, oranges, peaches, broccoli and green beans. There is some evidence to suggest that it can be as effective as certain antibiotics when treating UTIs, and it is thought that it works in a similar way to cranberry as it inhibits bacterial adherence to the urinary tract mucosa by attaching to the bacteria instead. For prevention, up to 2 g can be taken daily. In an acute infection you may want to take as much as 1 g three times daily for up to two weeks. However, caution should be applied if you are diabetic, even if your blood sugar levels are controlled. D-mannose is a sugar and can affect your blood sugar level.

A note on UTIs

I need to stress that if you have an active infection and it is not improving within a couple of days or getting worse, you need to go and see a GP as well as consulting with a herbal practitioner (for longer-term prevention strategies). If not adequately treated, this could progress further up the urinary tract to affect the bladder and the kidneys, and could be dangerous. Please don't ignore it (although it is normally quite difficult to ignore!).

Other lifestyle considerations

Hygiene, clothing and toilet paper

As we have already discovered, the vagina is self-cleaning, and unless you are trying anything self-directed from these pages or something recommended by a qualified health professional it doesn't need washing, not even with plain water, and certainly not with any soaps or gels. The labia can be washed with water, but not soap, but the mons (the fatty layer covering the labia that's covered in hair), can be washed as you would wash any other part of your body.

You may be asking, but what about those washes that have been specifically marketed for intimate hygiene? Well, all soaps, including those called intimate washes and especially fragranced ones, have the potential to knock our intimate pH and vaginal microbiome out, which can cause mild itching and could of course lead to thrush and bacterial vaginosis. It's worth remembering that it's entirely normal for vaginas and vulvas to have a smell—normally a light musky scent. It's only when that smell changes significantly to a foul, fishy or yeasty smell that it becomes a sign that something is wrong. Your smell may change over the month or over time too, and that is entirely normal. Why not become an expert at noticing when your natural smell slightly changes. Maybe you can even detect smells reminiscent of the food you've recently eaten. If you can, that's totally normal too!

When it comes to clothing, it's likely you already know that generally vaginas and vulvas are happier when we wear natural fibre underwear such as cotton, and even better, bamboo—which allows air to circulate, allowing our intimate areas to breathe, wicking away moisture, thus minimising the damp environment. A natural and, if possible, organic, cotton or bamboo cloth is also non-irritant to the skin. If you are prone to recurrent issues it would also benefit you to avoid tight-fitting clothing such as leggings or skinny jeans, which don't allow air to the area, and can impede a healthy circulation.

If you like cotton underwear, then you're going to love bamboo! Natural bamboo underwear, period wear and toilet paper can be a total revolution for irritated vaginas. Bamboo fibres wick away moisture very efficiently, can be made naturally from a fast-growing natural resource—and the thing I like about it the most is that it makes the most amazing toilet paper.

Believe it or not the fine dust from regular loo roll can irritate the vulval mucous membranes and there have even been studies about it.

Sometimes I will get a patient who tells me that they think they are crazy but think that their loo roll is making things worse. They are so relieved when I tell them that it's absolutely possible and, not only that, but likely. The amazing thing about bamboo toilet roll is that it doesn't really have that fine dust associated with regular toilet paper and therefore doesn't cause the irritation that wood-based toilet paper does. Making changes like this can rapidly provide a level of comfort, minimising repeated irritation, while your other changes and remedies can start to take effect. Check the Resources section for some great bamboo brands. Another hygiene tip is to make sure that you wipe front to back after urinating. But you knew that already, right?!

Some considerations for pubic hair

Possibly political, conceivably cultural and an imaginative way of self-expression, pubic hair can be a matter of embarrassment or pride, upkeep or a non-issue. Evolutionarily pubic hair is there as an attempt at first line defence against things we don't want near the vagina, but I have known women who chose to remove it for comfort, if irritation or excess heat and damp have been an issue, and women who have chosen to keep it or trim it for the same reasons. There is no hard and fast rules for pubic hair when it comes to vaginal health: use your experience to inform your preferences when finding out what's best for you.

Periodwear

Periodwear, menstrual wear, whatever we want to call it (just don't call it 'feminine hygiene', pleeease) we are living in amazing times. We now have more options than any other women at any other time in history to find a solution that fits us!! First things first, all of our preferences are different for this. Some of us won't like using tampons (hand up here!), some of us can't stand pads, and some of us need to wear both on certain days.

Some of the options we now have include:

- Traditional disposable pads
- Traditional disposable tampons
- Tampons with reusable applicators
- CBD-soaked tampons
- Organic pads and tampons
- Menstrual cups

- Period underwear including bamboo options (see the Resources section)
- Flex Menstrual Discs
- Reusable pads

And with such a great selection we can really rethink our choices to make sure they are working for us.

First of all, what's 'wrong' with the traditional options, and why might they not be serving you (or the planet). Well, apart from disposables not being an ecological choice, they may contain plastics, chemicals such as dioxin, pesticides and propylene glycol, which can disrupt hormones,[64] and dyes or fragrance which can not only get into the bloodstream and disrupt hormones but can cause vaginal and vulval irritation.

To minimise disruption to your intimate ecology here are a few top tips when considering your options:

- Choose something organic and wickable (wickable means that any moisture is allowed to easily evaporate rather than staying trapped against your skin, keeping the area damp).
- If you like something insertable, try switching from tampons to cups, and make sure you keep up with the cleaning routine recommended by the manufacturer (which is very easy to do). However, if you are experiencing vaginal irritation, insertable options may not be the best choice for you while you sort the situation out.
- If you go for reusable, make sure you boil wash and change every 6–12 months to reduce the likelihood of bacteria build-up, which might contribute to tipping your vaginal ecology out if you're susceptible.

I've included some links to good manufacturers in the Resources section, but this is only a selection—there are many more and new ones are coming on the market all the time.

Rowing and cycling

As previously mentioned, avid cyclists and rowers may find they get intimate irritation from chaffing on long rides or rows. Anti-chaffing chamois or 'shammy' creams are marketed for this but often they don't have very vulva-friendly ingredients, which may rather contribute to any irritation experienced. Instead, see lubricants in Resources section (p. 188) for some viable alternatives.

Low histamine diet

Sometimes, when everything else has been ruled out and vaginal issues are recurring, it can be worth considering histamine intolerance. Histamine is found in all tissues of the body and in many foods and herbs. We have histamine receptors throughout our bodies. Not only is histamine released in allergy and injury to bring immune system components to the affected site, but it is also involved in a variety of muscle contractions and in the stimulation of gastric acid secretion.

People with low levels of an enzyme called diamine oxidase, which helps break down histamine, may experience histamine intolerance which can look a lot like hay fever: irritation of the mucosal membranes, hives, itchy or flushed skin, red eyes, streaming eyes and nose, facial swelling and irritation of the vaginal mucosa. It can also cause a drop in blood pressure, headaches or migraines, nausea, heart palpitations, anxiety or a panic attack.

Histamine intolerance is specifically a reaction to an overload of histamines in the body, rather than a histaminic reaction to other allergens. Treatment may involve reducing histamine-containing foods from the diet such as cheeses, yoghurt, kefir, sauerkraut, processed meats, canned and pickled foods, smoked meats, vinegars, alcoholic drinks, avocado, chickpeas, lentils, strawberries, citrus fruits, chocolate, cashews, walnuts, tomatoes, bananas, aubergines, spinach, wheat germ and papaya. This may feel overwhelming but may just be the key if everything else has been ruled out. If you suspect this might be the key based on your symptoms, look for a practitioner specialising in histamine intolerance to help you.

Dietary impacts on digestive health

As we've discussed above, good digestive health can benefit vaginal health. Abdominal congestion and a sluggish digestion can impact on immune health and waste clearance in the area and can influence the hepatic recirculation of oestrogens. This will have a knock-on effect for vaginal health. If you're emptying your bowels less than once a day or you experience some discomfort passing your stools, you might want to look at hydration levels, dietary fibre levels and employ some of the tactics discussed in the digestion section.

Dietary impacts on immune health

For so many vaginal health issues, the immune system is either implicated, or at least plays a role in how it deals with the overgrowth of a particular set of microbes, or in the over-activity and dysregulation of an immune condition. We can influence our immune health with herbs and the food that we eat. In order to optimise our immune health, we may want to reduce refined sugars, trans-fats, alcohol and processed foods. A good rule of thumb is that when buying pre-prepared food of any type, the longer the list of ingredients is, and the less recognisable the ingredients are, the less of it you should be eating.

Organic foods, which have fewer pesticide residues, while being grown in soil with better nutrition, often have higher levels of vitamins and trace elements in them that are required by our body to function at an optimal level. Let's make every bite work for us, calorie by calorie. Try to make sure that you 'eat the rainbow' each day. That is, eating fresh foods from each of the colour groups to ensure you are getting a good nutritional range.

When it comes to vegetarian or vegan diets, it's worth making sure that you are getting enough B vitamins from your food. For example, one patient I saw suffered from recurrent thrush until she started eating meat after years of being vegan. If you decide to eat meat, make sure you eat organic to ensure welfare standards, as well as reducing pollutants such as antibiotics and other medicines or chemicals that the animal has stored in its fats (this is where mammals store any substances that their bodies cannot process). For specific concerns and individualised dietary advice, speak with your medical herbalist or nutritional therapist.

Vaginal dilators

If vaginismus is an issue for you, dilator sets are effective tools that can help you override involuntary vaginal and pelvic floor contractions. Work with a pelvic physiotherapist to help you get the best from this and other sensitive and relevant exercises. Dilators are also helpful for those with a neo-vagina to help ensure the maintenance of the new structure.

Blood glucose levels and how to go sugar-free or low-sugar, if you want to

Ever felt 'hangry' or noticed your energy levels dip in the afternoon (and any other time)? Chances are you are experiencing the highs and lows of not having a well-balanced blood sugar/glucose level. While this can be a prelude to a pre-diabetic warning, your body is also giving you information that, if you listen to it, can help you.

I don't believe there have been any studies that have proved a link between sugar consumption and VVC, although I have seen it empirically plenty of times in my clinic. The theory is that having excess sugar in the diet contributes to greater levels of sugar in the blood than needed, proving a wonderful food source for the *Candida* spp.

Eating a diet that contains lots of sugary snacks and hidden sugars and then having a recurrent or chronic form of VVC can be a sign that your Blood Glucose Level is out of balance. Because of the type of food you are consuming, you get a rush of sugar into your system. Your body employs insulin and other factors to try and reduce the level of sugar dumped into the blood and then, because it's had to deploy all of its tools rather enthusiastically to deal with it, your energy suddenly drops off as there isn't enough sugar available in the bloodstream. Automatically you reach for another sugary or simple carbohydrate snack to make you feel better. As you can see it swings from one extreme to the other.

If this is relevant for you, balance your blood sugar levels by finding ways to reduce excess sugars in your diet. Adding a small amount of protein (nuts, nut butters, seeds and pulses can be great options) alongside your carbohydrate intake has been shown to slow down the rate of sugar entering the bloodstream to make it more sustainable and manageable. If you are suffering from RVVC and CVVC and you notice a correlation with sugar intake you might want to think about quitting refined excess sugars altogether. It's a big decision, but your body will undoubtedly thank you.

Here are some tips:

– **No one said this was going to be easy:** it has been said that sugar is eight times more addictive than cocaine—we are evolutionarily programmed to crave it! You need to be aware of this and *be prepared!*
– **But the reassuring and good news is:** it's totally possible and many people have trodden the path that you are now preparing to tread! Not only is it doable, but in most cases, within a few weeks of quitting, you will no longer crave sugar or sugary foods, and if you do have something, you will be shocked and surprised at just how sweet it is! Be prepared to feel free!
– **What are the benefits of quitting sugar? Why is it for me?** Well, I guess we are here because some of the symptoms that you are experiencing are being exacerbated or triggered by sugar. Some of the benefits of having a no-refined-sugar diet will be: balanced blood

sugar levels meaning fewer energy dips, mood swings, and shakiness; less triggering of things like eczema, thrush and oral thrush; and a reduced chance of developing type II diabetes. But there are many more. Refined sugar has even been linked to tumour growth and inflammation! Eating sugar means you are consuming empty calories—you're getting no nutritional benefit at all—your recommended calorie intake could be working much harder for you! The benefits are many.

– **What to expect and how do you do it?** Often we crave a sweet food when we are not hungry. Although eating a healthy meal or snack and eating a sweet food both involve the same action, i.e. eating, essentially they are triggered by different desires (e.g. hunger vs craving a sugar 'reward/hit'), so breaking the association between food and sugar is important. While our body needs carbohydrates to produce energy, complex carbohydrates that release energy in a slow and sustained way (such as brown rice, sweet potato, or other low GI/GL foods) are the best way to go. Sugar is a simple carbohydrate and dumps all the energy into your bloodstream in one hit—thereby producing the mood swings etc.

When giving up refined sugars it is entirely normal for you to still crave sugar for a good couple of weeks—it may even make you feel angry, irritable, possibly even depressed, or you may experience headaches (as your body 'detoxes'), but once you have broken that craving, the only way is up! So don't give up! It may seem that it is just about cutting out obvious sugary foods (cakes, biscuits, sweets, sugar in teas and coffees), but there is also an extraordinary amount of hidden sugar in everyday foods you may not have even have thought of, so always read the packet and make the non-sugar choices.

To start with, it may be easier to prepare all your food at home from scratch, to ensure it is sugar-free, but as you move forwards you will get to know what is 'sugar-free' and can be bought when you are out. The good news is, as a society we are now more switched on to low-sugar foods, so these choices are easier to find and make—plus there are loads of good 'no-sugar' recipe books out there.

– **A word about food choices:** as well as actively choosing no-sugar foods, it's also worth looking at low GI/GL ingredients. These are foods that have a low glycemic index or load, which measures the amount of 'naturally occurring' sugars that are in the food and how quickly that is released into the blood. The lower the number, the more stable the release is, and the better it is at maintaining sustained energy release. This is great!

Another tip I have relates to weaning yourself away from sugar when craving a hit. When this happens, acknowledge what is happening and that your body is not necessarily hungry but is looking for that sugar 'reward'. Then replace that reward with a no-sugar substitute (I have found an oat cake helpful, but others may find a handful of raw veg works). Because you are giving this reward via the same 'route', i.e. by eating, it can go some way to 'tricking' the body that it is getting the reward it desires—I'm not saying it will be the same, but just that it may help.

- **Sugar substitutes:** you may have seen lots of sugar substitutes available in the shops—xylitol, agave syrup, coconut sugar, artificial sweeteners (these artificial sweeteners are very hard on the liver and never recommended!), the list goes on. These alternatives may be considered healthier than sugar (putting aside any ecological considerations). However, because the body does not often digest them, passing out the other end untouched, they don't help reduce that craving for a sugar hit—they still stimulate the sweet taste buds and so they do nothing to actually help you quit. Best to avoid them.

   Honey is perhaps a little different because while it is packed with unrefined sugars, it also contains many other beneficial properties, so let's not write it off altogether—but just avoid it for now.

- **Alcohol:** the sad fact is that all alcohol breaks down into sugars in the body. While following a no-refined-sugar lifestyle I am recommending that this also includes no alcohol.

- **Supportive supplements:** chromium supplements can be useful to support you during your no-sugar journey—they help your body to utilise insulin and balance your blood sugar level. A general recommended daily dose is 200µg or lower and is taken with food (foods high in vitamin C increase its absorption) or a glass of water. You can find these supplements also combined with cinnamon which is fine. Chromium can also be found in whole grain cereals, potatoes, peanut butter, nuts and seafood.

- **A word about fruit:** to start with, it may also be helpful to remove fruit from your diet. However, and this is important to note: *this should only ever be for a short period of time (2–3 weeks), and plenty of fresh vegetables should be eaten to make sure you are still getting your*

5 *(minimum) a day.* I am in no way advocating a no-fruit lifestyle, and when you reintroduce fruit (after three weeks max) there are some smart choices that you can make to ensure you are able to maintain your low-sugar approach.

Essentially, anything that tastes super sweet probably is. There are some great fruits that you can still eat, such as berries (all, apart from strawberries—they are super sweet so save for a special occasion—however other berries are all fine and so good for you!), kiwi, pineapple, citrus fruits, and nectarines. Bananas are generally a no-no (but please ensure that you maintain adequate levels of potassium in your diet elsewhere, especially if you are on any standard allopathic diuretics)—as well as dates, prunes, grapes and raisins. This also applies to fruit juices.

If you need support or guidance then please find a qualified practitioner who has relevant experience to help you.

Journaling prompts

While we are aware that vaginal health can impact our emotional and mental health, it seems as though our mental and emotional health can also affect our vaginal health. Have you ever felt that too? This an area where research is needed (but how would one even go about designing that?!), but on a human level it would make sense that a place that is so connected with our emotions (think sexual encounters and childbirth) would have this feedback loop with our emotional, mental and spiritual health.

If recurrent vaginal and vulval issues affect you, it would be worth spending some time journaling about them, and your mental, emotional and spiritual health. Not only will it help you to connect more deeply to your body, possibly gaining an innate understanding of what it needs and what you need, but it may help you find any emotional or mental roots linked to your physical health. Journaling can be a great way of bringing the unconscious to our conscious awareness, and if you like, it can be done as a form of a stream of consciousness writing, or bullet points.

The following are some journal prompts you can use to start the dialogue with yourself. Allow your responses to inform further enquiry and exploration.

- How do I feel about my intimate health?
- How do I feel about any restrictions it is placing on me?
- How is my health issue serving me?
- What messages could my body be trying to tell me? (You totally have permission to be as 'creative' or as out there as you like.)
- If my vagina could speak, what would she say she needed?
- What would you tell your vagina if you could?
- What is the earliest root cause of my recurrent issues? (These root causes don't necessarily need to be physical, they can also be emotional, mental, spiritual, traumatic or a combination.)
- What first step could I take to help me heal my root cause?

The big thing here is not to judge anything that comes up for you. When you read it back it may not make sense. All answers are welcome here, and journaling regularly over time can be a great way to start seeing patterns and themes that come up for you. It is useful information for you and another piece of the puzzle.

Singing?

You may find that experimenting with singing can be a way to connect to your vagina, and the messages she is trying to give you or the creative power she has. I have heard of singing teachers suggesting that their clients should try 'singing through their vaginas' (not literally of course) to really help them engage in that energy we naturally have there, and this could be a lovely way to give voice to your vagina and her message if you feel moved to do so. I've also heard from a somatic therapist that if someone is residing in their pelvis, they find their voice …

Other creative expression

If connecting in with the energetic centre of your vagina seems hard or blocked in some way, you could try experimenting with other creative expressions to find a way in. These could have the aim of trying to feel your way through, to vent, or to create a vital expression of you in that moment. Perfection is not the aim, so don't self-censor, and you don't need to show anyone unless you want to. The value is in the act itself and you may find it a good way to get that creative power portal energy flowing. Ideas include, but aren't limited to:

- action painting
- body painting
- other types painting, drawing or mark-making
- pottery and glass work
- music making
- DJ/VJing
- photography
- cooking
- primal screaming
- gardening
- interior design
- knitting/crochet
- sculpture
- print making
- collage
- drama
- creative writing
- storytelling
- dancing
- flower arranging
- swimming even

Whatever feels connected and good to you. It's just gives us the opportunity for a different way in, one perhaps that doesn't get too tied in knots with our cognitive filtering process, our monkey mind. Go with the flow, try it out and see what happens. You might get inspired, but don't worry if not. Everyone has their own way to connect. It's just a case of finding your key.

Pelvic/women's health physio

I've mentioned pelvic or women's health physios quite a number of times throughout the book. There are physiotherapists that specialise in, you guessed it, the female pelvic bowl and surrounding structures. They can be helpful postnatally, in pregnancy, prolapse, vaginal dryness, sexual discomfort, constipation, incontinence, chronic pelvic pain and lower back pain to name a few, and can take a key role in supporting you. Check the Resources section for their professional organisations, to help you find a practitioner should you wish to.

Guided mediation to help your connection with your vagina

If you've had a long and painful road with vaginal irritation of any sort you can start to feel a disconnection from that part of yourself. You're so fed up with it that it starts by not wanting to think about that place; by pretending it's not happening; by taking your attention away from it to elsewhere. Then you stop mentally inhabiting that part of your body. It then leads to numbing that part of yourself and perhaps to a total disconnect between you and your sexual energy and feminine self. I know because I've been there. It's totally understandable to feel this way, but as 21st-century women it's not what we want and we definitely deserve more. We deserve to get to a position where we can start to reawaken play.

Alongside any herbal products, herbal medicines, bodywork, dietary interventions or allopathic medicines you might be taking, caring for your mental health and psyche is unbelievably important and can be a missing link—to do this work puts you back in touch with your body and reawakens play. In order to help, I developed the following meditation that you can use to begin that journey back to yourself. (An audio version is available from my website).

Start by finding some quiet time and space for yourself—around ten minutes would be perfect—in a comfortable place to lay down, with a pillow under your head and one under your knees, as this allows your belly to soften and relax. Close your eyes and allow yourself to breathe deeply for several breaths. Feel the points of contact between your body and the ground; feel the earth supporting your body. On each inhale, feel the air expanding in your chest and lungs, and on exhaling through your mouth, allow your shoulders to soften and relax as you feel any tension leaving your body.

After resting here for several breaths, place your hands flat on your belly below your belly button, with thumbs and fingertips touching, creating a heart shape over your intimate area. This is the seat of your feminine power. As you continue to take mindful breaths, breathe in and visualise that you are inhaling a beautiful gold or rose coloured light. It fills your lungs and travels down through your heart. And on the out-breath, it travels back up as you breathe out through your mouth. On your next in-breath you feel that light travelling down from your lungs, into your heart space and right down into your vagina.

As you breathe out, visualise the breath-light coming back up through your vagina and your heart and then out again, all the time visualising this beautiful gold or rose light filling your heart and vagina. Carry on for as long as you feel comfortable, creating a circuit of breath-light, almost like a figure of 8 or the infinity symbol, relaxing into the practice and feeling your heart-vagina connection. This rose or gold light symbolises love and you are sending love, light and a feeling of safety from your heart down to your vagina and back again.

When you are ready to end, bring yourself back to the room by becoming aware of any sounds or smells in the room, then wiggle your fingers and toes and maybe have a stretch and when you are ready open your eyes, thanking yourself for being present. You may want to spend a few minutes journaling about your experience—did you feel a connection? Did any emotions or messages come up for you? Did you feel any resistance?

Anything you feel is valid. Don't worry if you don't feel a connection the first time. It can take a few attempts before you really feel it. Stick with the practice as often as you like and see how you go. Journaling, as above, can help you to record any progress or patterns that come up for you.

There are other therapeutics practitioners can use (not mentioned in this book)

And so, we come close to the end of this book. I hope you've found lots of tools to help you here on your journey. I really want to emphasise that if anything from the Limitations section are going on for you or you are not noticing a change or reduction in your symptoms within a month's time, then it really would be in your best interests to go and see a qualified practitioner who can help you.

The benefits of seeing a practitioner are that they have a greater level of experience and understanding of how to best help you, a full knowledge of all safety aspects they need to take into account, as well as several therapeutic options not covered here, as they can only be obtained and prescribed by qualified practitioners.

I really want to encourage you to seek out their help. After all, that's what we're trained to do!

This woman's work

If the vagina could make an animal noise it would be a lion's roar.

– Natasha Richardson

So, after all this, why do I care about vaginal health so much and why is it important? Aside from the comfort and health issues, what makes this bigger than just the personal, and why have I dedicated my career to it? Looking at the title of this book might give some clues. I believe the vagina and associated structures to be an energetic power centre, the power portal. Often seen as mysterious, but always, in actual fact, essential. Not just the centre of sexual power and sensuality, but a source of feminine and creative energy, I truly believe our power portals have been subjugated and silenced for long enough.

While women's health is starting to be truly foregrounded, taking the place it deserves, vaginal health is so often still the missing piece, the one place still considered too taboo to go. And if you have first-hand experience of how debilitating a vaginal health issue can be, and how hard it is to get allopathic medicine to take seriously, diagnose and treat, you know how much it can curb our expressions' in the world. Let's take some of that power back.

I truly believe that the world needs more feminine power, creativity and leadership, and it is my hope that through healing our own, and society's, relationship with the vagina, whose name is so often dared not spoken, we can have a greater impact for good in the work we create, do and embody. For me it's about making, and helping others to make, empowered, informed choices, and creating my own expressions in the world. Wylde work indeed.

What will you create?

PART FIVE

MATERIALS

GLOSSARY

I've used a few 'medical' words in this book. This isn't to confuse, but because they most elegantly and accurately describe some of the concepts I am conveying—they are simply the best words for the situation. In addition to this, I have used this medical terminology because I don't believe that medical vocabulary should be some sort of secretive language, reserved only for those in the 'know', in white coats. I believe very much in the democratisation of medicine, and knowledge of our bodies, and so here is a glossary to help explain the concepts behind the terms I have used.

Allopathic	conventional medicine.
Alterative	a herb that is known as a blood and lymph cleanser and promote the renewal of body tissue.
Anterior	relating to the front of the body.
Amphoteric	having two opposing characteristics that express dynamic balance.
Astringent	a substance that binds to and constricts human tissues on contact.
Atrophy	decreasing in size of an organ, cell, muscle or other tissue, from a normal size to something smaller.

AV	aerobic vaginitis.
Bioavailable	the degree to which a substance is available for absorption into the body.
BV	bacterial vaginosis.
Colposcopy	the procedure of examining the cervix, vagina and vulva with a magnifying instrument that has a light attached called a colposcope.
Congenital	something you were born with.
CV	cytolytic vaginosis.
CVVC	chronic vulvovaginal candidiasis.
Dysbiosis	an imbalance in a microbiome that results in harmful species having dominance.
Empirical	based on, or verifiable by, observation and experience.
Endogenous	originating from within the body.
Eubiotic/eubiosis	an optimal balance of microflora.
Excipient	an inactive substance that serves as the vehicle or medium for a drug or other active substance.
Exogenous	originating from outside the body.
Galactagogue	a substance that promotes milk production in humans.
Homeostasis	a state of dynamic balance in the body systems required for maintenance and functionality. This is maintained by constant adjustment of the biochemical and physiological pathways.
Iatrogenic	relating to illness caused by medical intervention.
Innervation	the distribution and supply of nerves to an organ or body part.
Leucorrhea	a white vaginal discharge. It might be normal or it might indicate infection, inflammation or congestion of the vaginal mucous membranes.
Marc	herb material used to make a tincture.
Menstruum	the liquid portion used to make a tincture.
Mediation	the act of acting as an intermediary between two biological processes within the body.
Nociception	the perception of painful stimuli.
Oophorectomy	surgical removal of the ovaries.
Os	opening.

Peristalsis	a series of wavelike muscle contractions that move the food through the digestive tract.
Phase	referring to the oil-based or water-based ingredients of a topical application.
Posterior	relating to the rear of the body.
Potentiate	the effect of increasing the potency or effectiveness of a treatment.
RVVC	recurrent vulvovaginal candidiasis.
A Simple	a herbal preparation containing one herb.
Somatise	the expression of psychological symptoms by the body.
Systemic	something which affects or exerts its action on the whole of the human system/body.
Thymoleptic	a substance that modulates a person's mood, normally for the better.
VVC	vulvovaginal candidiasis.

RESOURCES (ALL CORRECT AT TIME OF GOING TO PRINT)

Condoms

Lelo Hex https://www.lelohex.com
Hanx https://www.hanxofficial.com
Fair Squared https://www.fairsquared.com/en/products/condoms/
Skyn https://www.skynfeel.co.uk
EXS https://exscondoms.com

Dental dams

Lorals Pants https://mylorals.com
Sheer Glyde Dams https://glydehealth.com/products/sheer-glyde-dams/

Sexual health screening

IplaySafe https://www.iplaysafe.app
Free testing in the UK https://sh24.org.uk

Glass, ceramic and body-safe crystal dildos

Fine Bone – porcelain pleasure tools https://www.finebone.co.uk
Onna Lifestyle https://www.onnalifestyle.com
Chakrubs https://www.chakrubs.com

Other pleasure tools

Dame https://www.dameproducts.com
Layla Martin – for great resources https://laylamartin.com

Intimate lubricants

Into the Wylde https://intothewylde.com
Sylk https://sylk.co.uk

Vibrating dilators for vaginismus

Sh! Emporium https://www.sh-womenstore.com/sh-vibrating-sili-cone-vaginismus-set.html

Professional practitioner bodies (for finding registered practitioners in different disciplines)

Medical herbalists

The National Institute of Medical Herbalists
The College of Practitioners of Phytotherapy
Association of Master Herbalists
Unified Register of Herbal Practitioners
American Herbalists Guild

Naturopaths

General Council and Register of Naturopaths
British Naturopathic Association
Association of Naturopathic Practitioners

Nutritional therapists

British Association of Nutritional Therapists
Institute of Optimum Nutrition

Somatic and sexual therapists

The Association of Somatic & Integrative Sexologists
College of Sexual and Relationship Therapists

Psychological therapies

British Association for Counselling and Psychotherapy
UK Council for Psychotherapy
United Kingdom Register of Counsellors and Psychotherapists
Rapid Transformational Therapy

Abdominal massage therapies

Mizan Therapy
The Arvigo Institute
Fertility Massage

Pelvic health physiotherapists

Pelvic Obstetric and Gynaecological Physiotherapy
The Pelvic Health Society
Fertility Massage Therapy

Further help for people with cervical screenings

https://www.nhs.uk/conditions/cervical-screening/further-help-and-support/

Great herb stockists in the UK

Neals Yard Remedies
Baldwins
Dee Atkinson

Botanica Medica
Apotheca Natural Health
Invivo Healthcare
Caley's Apothecary

Supplements and products for self-guided purchase

Invivo Healthcare – many amazing therapeutics and diagnostics for various microbiome sites. In particular their Bio.Me Femme range https://invivohealthcare.com
Pukka Herbs – they do a great mushroom supplement called Mushroom Gold https://www.pukkaherbs.com/uk/en/
Mushrooms – MycoNutri https://myconutri.com
Better You – transdermal and oral spray vitamins https://betteryou.com
Optibac – for probiotics https://www.optibacprobiotics.com
Cheeky Panda – bamboo toilet paper https://uk.cheekypanda.com
Boody – bamboo underwear https://boody.co.uk

Menstrual wear selection (many other brands exist)

Period pants

Modibody https://www.modibodi.co.uk
Bamboo period pants – The Bamboo House https://the-bamboo-house.co.uk/collections/period-underwear
Bamboo period pants – Intimya https://www.intimya.co.uk

Sustainable organic disposables

TOTM https://www.totm.com
Naturacare https://www.natracare.com
Yoni https://yoni.care
&Sisters https://andsisters.com

Discs and cups

Flex https://flexfits.uk
Nixit https://nixit.com

Mooncup https://www.mooncup.co.uk
Allmatters https://www.allmatters.com
Lunette https://uk.lunette.com
Intimina https://intimina.com
&Sisters https://andsisters.com

CBD infused

Daye https://yourdaye.com

Reusable cloth pads (including bamboo)

Nora & Bloom https://www.bloomandnora.com
Bambaw https://bambaw.com

Charities working to prevent FGM

https://www.orchidproject.org
http://www.fgmnationalgroup.org
https://bit.ly/3oPb1GU
https://www.freedomcharity.org.uk/what-we-do/female-genital-mutilation/
https://www.savethechildren.org.uk/what-we-do/health/fgm

Recommended reading

The Vagina: A Literary and Cultural History by Emma L. E. Rees
The Vagina Bible: The Vulva And The Vagina – Separating the Myth from the Medicine by Dr Jen Gunter
Threads by Lisa January
Wild Power: Discover the Magic of Your Menstrual Cycle and Awaken the Feminine Path to Power by Alexandra Pope and Sjanie Hugo Wurlitzer
Informed. Aware. Empowered: A Self-Guided Journey to Clear Paps by Denell Barbara Nawrocki
When the Body Says No: The Hidden Cost of Stress by Gabor Maté

And finally ... just a selection of the great and relevant therapists I know

Jo Farren – medical herbalist, doula and breastfeeding peer supporter

Andrea Balboni (Lush Coaching) – relationships and sex coach

Natasha Richardson (Forage Botanicals) – natural answers for period pain

Moira Bradfield (Intimate Ecology) – one of my teachers and a naturopath specialising in vaginal health

Kate Waters – nutritional therapists, very experienced in vaginal health

Inna Duckworth – medical herbalist & nutritional therapist, working with overall female wellbeing, fertility and vaginal health

Kat Hesse – medical herbalist, mind-body health, yoga, chi gong, feldenkrais, pilates, and somatic movement therapist, working with vaginal health, low libido and pelvic floor health

Kathie Bishop (The Wylde Herbalist) – that's me!

REFERENCES

1. World Health Organization, 'Female Genital Mutilation' (2020). https://www.who.int/news-room/fact-sheets/detail/female-genital-mutilation (Accessed 15 March 2021).
2. Jen Gunter, *The Vagina Bible: The Vulva and the Vagina—Separating the Myth from the Medicine* (London: Piatkus, 2019).
3. S. Winston, *Women's Anatomy of Arousal: Secret Maps to Buried Pleasure* (Kingston: Mango Garden, 2010).
4. The Establishment, 'The Insidious Reasons Doctors Are Botching Labiaplasties'. https://theestablishment.co/the-insidious-reasons-doctors-are-botching-labiaplasties/ (Accessed 27 August 2020).
5. Monique Brouillette, 'Decoding the Vaginal Microbiome'. *Scientific American*. https://www.scientificamerican.com/article/decoding-the-vaginal-microbiome/ (Accessed 9 May 2020).
6. Roxana J. Hickey, Xia Zhou, Jacob D. Pierson, Jacques Ravel and Larry J. Forney, 'Understanding Vaginal Microbiome Complexity from an Ecological Perspective'. *Translational Research*, Volume 160, Issue 4 (2012), pp. 267–282. doi: 10.1016/j.trsl.2012.02.008 (Accessed 9 May 2021).
7. Jacques Ravel, Pawel Gajer, Zaid Abdo, G. Maria Schneider, Sara S. K. Koenig, Stacey L. McCulle, Shara Karlebach, Reshma Gorle,

Jennifer Russell, Carol O. Tacket, Rebecca M. Brotman, Catherine C. Davis, Kevin Ault, Ligia Peralta and Larry J. Forney, 'Vaginal Microbiome of Reproductive-Age Women'. *Proceedings of the National Academy of Sciences*, Volume 108 (Supplement 1), (2011), pp. 4680–4687. doi: 10.1073/pnas.1002611107 (Accessed 9 May 2021).

8. L. L. Bradford and J. Ravel, 'The vaginal Mycobiome: A Contemporary Perspective in Fungi in Women's Health and Diseases'. *Virulence*, Volume 8, Issue 3 (2017), pp. 342–351. doi: 10.1080/21505594.2016.1237332 (Accessed 9 May 2021).

9. A. Goldstein, C. Pukall and I. Goldstein, *When Sex Hurts: A Woman's Guide to Banishing Sexual Pain.* 1st ed (Philadelphia: DeCapo Press, 2011).

10. A. Kölle, F.-A. Taran, K. Rall, D. Schöller, D. Wallwiener and S. Y. Brucker, 'Neovagina Creation Methods and their Potential Impact on Subsequent Uterus Transplantation: A Review'. *BJOG*, Volume 126, Issue 11 (2019), pp. 13–281335. (Accessed 27 August 2020).

11. M. Bradfield, 'Paediatrics: The Vaginal Microbiome in Childhood'. https://intimate-ecology-practitioner-training.teachable.com/courses/482320/lectures/8880512 (Accessed 27 August 2020).

12. Y. R. Smith, D. R. Berman and H. Quinch, 'Premenarchal Vaginal Discharge: Findings of Procedures to Rule Out Foreign Bodies'. *J. Pediatr. Adolesc. Gynecol.*, Volume 15, Issue 4 (2002), pp. 227–230. doi: 10.1016/s1083-3188(02)00160-2 (Accessed 9 May 2021).

13. R. Ashton and B. Leppard, *Differential Diagnosis in Dermatology.* 3rd ed (Abingdon: Radcliffe Publishing Ltd, 2005).

14. Roxana J. Hickey, Xia Zhou, Matthew L. Settles, Julie Erb, Kristin Malone, Melanie A. Hansmann, Marcia L. Shew, Barbara Van Der Pol, J. Dennis Fortenberry and Larry J. Forney, 'Vaginal Microbiota of Adolescent Girls Prior to the Onset of Menarche Resemble Those of Reproductive-Age Women' *mBio*, Volume 6, Issue 2 (2015), pp. e00097–15; doi: 10.1128/mBio.00097-15 (Accessed 9 May 2021).

15. Mark Beers, Robert Porter, Thomas Jones, Justin Kaplan and Michael Berkwits, *The Merck Manual of Diagnosis and Therapy*, 18th ed (New Jersey: Merck Research Laboratories, 2006).

16. Blandine Calasi-Germain, *The Female Pelvis: Anatomy and Exercises* (Seattle: Eastland Press Inc, 2003).

17. Miranda Farage and Howard Maiback, 'Lifetime Changes in the Vulva and Vagina'. *Arch. Gynecol. Obstet.*, Issue 273 (2006), pp. 195–202. doi: 10.1007/s00404-005-0079-x (Accessed 27 August 2020).

18. T. J. Aguin, and J. D. Sobel, 'Vulvovaginal Candidiasis in Pregnancy'. *Curr. Infect. Dis. Rep.*, Volume 17, Issue 30 (2015). doi: 10.1007/s11908-015-0462-0 (Accessed 9 May 2021).

19. 'Microbirth'. https://microbirth.com (Accessed 3 March 2021).

20. R. Amatya, S. Bhattaral, P. K. Mandal, H. Tuladhar and B. M. Karki, 'Urinary Tract Infection in Vaginiti: A Condition Overlooked'. *Nepal Med. Coll. J.*, Volume 15 (2013), pp. 65–67. pmid: 24592798 (Accessed 9 May 2021).

21. Nicole M. Gilbert and Amanda L. Lewis, 'Covert pathogenesis: Transient Exposures to Microbes as Triggers of Disease'. *PLoS Pathog.*, Volume 15, Issue 3 (2019), p. e1007586. doi: 10.1371/journal. ppat.1007586 (Accessed 9 May 2021).

22. Tara Suchak, Jane Hussey, Manjit Takhar and James Bellringer, 'Postoperative Trans Women in Sexual Health Clinics: Managing Common Problems After Vaginoplasty'. *BMJ Sexual & Reproductive Health*, Volume 41, Issue 4 (2015), pp. 245–247. (Accessed 27 August 2020).

23. Rebecca M. Brotman, Xin He, Pawel Gajer et al., 'Association Between Cigarette Smoking and the Vaginal Microbiota: A Pilot Study'. *BMC Infect. Dis.*, Volume 14, Issue 471 (2014). (Accessed 27 August 2020).

24. Ingrid Freundt, Toon A. M. Toolenaar, Frans J. M. Huikeshoven, Hans Jeekel and Aat C. Drogendijk, 'Long-Term Psychosexual and Psychosocial Performance of Patients with a Sigmoid Neovagina'. *American Journal of Obstetrics and Gynecology*, Volume 169, Issue 5 (1993), pp. 1210–1214. ISSN: 0002-9378. (Accessed 27 August 2020).

25. R. C. J. Kanhai, 'Sensate Vagina Pedicled-Spot for Male-to-Female Transsexuals: The Experience in the First 50 Patients'. *Aesth. Plast. Surg.*, Volume 40, pp. 284–287 (2016). (Accessed 27 August 2020).

26. Gill Barham, 'Am I Menopausal?'. *Radiant Menopause*. https://www.radiantmenopause.com/blog/menopausalme (2019) (Accessed 27 August 2020).

27. Joanie Mercier, Mélanie Morin, Dina Zaki, Barbara Reicherzer, Marie-Claude Lemieux, Samir Khalifé and Chantale Dumoulin, 'Pelvic floor Muscle Training as a Treatment For Genitourinary Syndrome of T Menopause: A Single-Arm Feasibility Study'. *Maturitas*, Volume 125 (2019), pp. 57–62. doi: 10.1016/j.maturitas.2019.03.002 (Accessed 4 February 2021).

27a. B. Musicki, T. Liu, G. A. Lagoda, T. J. Bivalacqua, T. D. Strong, and A. L. Burnett, 'Endothelial Nitric Oxide Synthase Regulation in Female Genital Tract Structures'. *The Journal of Sexual Medicine*, Volume 6, Supplement 3 (S3PROCEEDINGS) (2009), pp. 247–253. doi: 10.1111/j.1743-6109.2008.01122.x (Accessed 19 May 2021).

28. Milly Evans, 'Why are STIs on the Rise in Older People?' *Patient*. https://patient.info/news-and-features/why-are-stis-on-the-rise-in-older-people (Accessed 27 August 2020).

29. Christopher Hedley and Non Shaw, *The Herbal Book of Making and Taking* (London: Aeon Books, 2020).

30. Joanne Barnes, Linda A. Anderson and J. David Phillipson, *Herbal Medicines*. 3rd ed (London: RPS Publishing, 2007).

31. Elisabeth Brooke, *A Woman's Book of Herbs* (London: The Women's Press Ltd, 1992).

32. Thomas Bartram, *Bartram's Encyclopaedia of Herbal Medicine* (London: Robinson, 1998).

33. Peter Bradley, *British Herbal Compendium, Volume 2* (Bournemouth: British Herbal Medicine Association, 2006).

34. R. F. Weis, and Volker Fintelmann, *Herbal Medicine. 2nd Edition, Revised and Expanded* (Stuttgart: Thieme, 2000).

35. Jiling Lin, 'Tea (*Camellia sinensis*)'. *Herb Rally*. https://www.herbrally.com/monographs/tea (Accessed 11 November 2020).

36. Rebecca M. Brotman, Xin He, Pawel Gajer, Doug Fadrosh, Eva Sharma, Emmanuel F. Mongodin, Jacques Ravel, Elbert D. Glover, and Jessica M. Rath, 'Association Between Cigarette Smoking and the Vaginal Microbiota: A Pilot Study'. *BMC Infectious Diseases*, Volume 14, Article 471 (2014). (Accessed 27 August 2020).

37. Martin Powell, *Medicinal Mushrooms: A Clinical Guide* (Ferndown: Mycology Press, 2012).

38. Francis Brinkler, *Herbal Contraindications and Drug Interactions*. 3rd ed (Oregon: Eclectic Medical Publications, 2001).

39. Peter Bradley, *British Herbal Compendium, Volume 1* (Bournemouth: British Herbal Medicine Association, 1992).

40. Jim Mann and Stewart Truswell (eds), *Essentials of Human Nutrition* (Oxford: Oxford University Press, 2007).

41. Goran Vujic, Alenka Jajac Knez, Vefrana Despot Stafanovic and Verdrana Kuzmic Vrbanovic, 'Efficacy of Orally Applied Probiotic Capsules for Bacterial vaginosis and Other Vaginal Infections: A Double-Blind, Randomized, Placebo-Controlled Study'. *Eur. J. Obstet. Gynecol. Reprod. Biol.*, Volume 168, Issue 1 (2013), pp. 75–79. doi: 10.1016/j.ejogrb.2012.12.031 (Accessed 27 August 2020).

42. Mariëlle A. J. Beerepoot, Gerben ter Riet, Sita Nys, Willem M. van der Wal, Corianne A. J. M. de Borgie, Theo M. de Reijke, Jan M. Prins, Jeanne Koeijers, Annelies Verbon, Ellen Stobberingh, Suzanne E. Geerlings, '*Lactobacilli* vs Antibiotics to Prevent Urinary Tract Infections: A Randomized, Double-blind, Noninferiority Trial in Postmenopausal Women'. *Archives of Internal Medicine*, Volume 172, Issue 9 (2012), pp. 704–711. doi: 10.1001/archinternmed.2012.777 (Accessed 27 August 2020).

43. R. C. R. Martinez, S. A. Franceschini, M. C. Patta, S. M. Quintana, R. C. Candido, J. C. Ferreira, E. C. P. De Martinis and G. Reid, 'Improved Treatment of Vulvovaginal Candidiasis with Fluconazole Plus Probiotic *Lactobacillus rhamnosus* GR-1 and *Lactobacillus reuteri* RC-14'. *Lett. Appl. Microbiol.*, Volume 48, Issue 3 (2009), pp. 269–274. doi: 10.1111/j.1472-765X.2008.02477.x (Epub 2 February 2009; Accessed 27 August 2020).

44. M. Yaralizadeh, P. Abedi, S. Najar, F. Manjoyan, A. Saki, 'Effect of *Foeniculum vulgare* (fennel) Vaginal Cream on Vaginal Atrophy in Postmenopausal Women: A Double-Blind Randomized Placebo-Controlled Trial'. *Maturitas*, Volume 84 (2016), pp. 75–80. doi: 10.1016/j.maturitas.2015.11.005 (Accessed 29 August 2021).

45. A. Gupta, N. K. Upadhyay, R. C. Sawhney and R. Kumar, 'A Poly-Herbal Formation Accelerates Normal and Impaired Diabetic Wound Healing'. *Wound Repair Regen.*, Volume 16, Issue 6 (2008), pp. 784–790. doi: 10.1111/j.1524-475X.2008.00431.x (Accessed 30 August 2020).

46. A. Gupta, R. Kumar, K. Pal, V. Singh, P. K. Banerjee and R. C. Sawhney, 'Influence of Sea Buckthorn (*Hippophae rhamnoides* L.) Flavone on Dermal Wind Healing in Rats'. *Mol. Cell. Biochem.*, Volume 290, Issues 1–2 (2006), pp. 193–198. doi: 10.1007/s11010-006-9187-6 (Accessed 30 August 2021).

47. Matthew Wood, *The Practice of Traditional Western Herbalism: Basic Doctrine, Energetics and Classification* (Berkeley: North Atlantic Books, 2004).

48. Emily Blake, 'Tending to our "Mycobiome"—Vaginal and Beyond'. *Invivo Healthcare*. https://invivohealthcare.com/education/articles/thrush-probiotic/?mc_cid=dfd1c7915b&mc_eid=655c78696a (Accessed 27 August 2020).

49. Matthew Wood, *The Earthwise Herbal: A Complete Guide to Old World Medicinal Plants* (Berkeley: North Atlantic Books, 2008).

50. Susun S. Weed, *Down There: Sexual and Reproductive Health—The Wise Woman Way* (Woodstock: Ashe Tree Publishing, 2011).
51. Association for the Advancement of Restorative Medicine. https://restorativemedicine.org/library/monographs/ashwagandha (Accessed 11 November 2020).
52. Charles M. Strom and Elliot M. Levine, 'Chronic Vaginal Candidiasis Responsive to Biotin Therapy in a Carrier of Biotinidase Deficiency'. *Obstetrics & Gynecology*, Volume 92, Issue 4, Part 2 (1998), pp. 644–646. (Accessed 12 November 2020).
53. Michael Tierra, 'For Many, an Effective Natural Approach for the Treatment of Mild States of Depression and Anxiety'. *Planet Herbs.* https://planetherbs.com/research-center/specific-herbs-articles/albizia-the-tree-of-happiness/ (Accessed 12 November 2020).
54. Adrian F. Gombart, 'The Vitamin D-Antimicrobial Peptide Pathway and its Role in Protection Against Infection'. *Future Microbiology*, Volume 4, Issue 9 (2009), pp. 1151–1165. doi: 10.2217/fmb.09.87 (Accessed 13 November 2020).
55. Duygu Övünç Hacıhamdioğlu, Demet Altun, Bülent Hacıhamdioğlu, Ferhat Çekmez, Gökhan Aydemir, Mustafa Kul, Tuba Müftüoglu, Selami Süleymanoglu and Ferhan Karademir (2016). 'The Association between Serum 25-Hydroxy Vitamin D Level and Urine Cathelicidin in Children with a Urinary Tract Infection'. *Journal of Clinical Research in Pediatric Endocrinology*, Volume 8, Issue 3 (2016), pp. 325–329. doi: 10.4274/jcrpe.2563 173 (Accessed 13 November 2020).
56. Christopher Hobbs, *Usnea: The Herbal Antibiotic and the Medicinal Lichens* (Capitola: Botanica Press, 1990).
57. Vladislav N. Krasnopolsky, Vera N. Prilepskaya, Franco Polatti, Nina V. Zarochentseva, Guldana R. Bayramova, Maurizio Caserini, and Renata Palmieri, 'Efficacy of Vitamin C Vaginal Tablets as Prophylaxis for Recurrent Bacterial vaginosis: A Randomised, Double-Blind, Placebo-Controlled Clinical Trial'. *Journal of Clinical Medicine Research*, Volume 5, Issue 4 (2013), pp. 309–315. doi: (Accessed 13 November 2020).
58. Jocelyn Anstey Watkins, Jonathan D. C. Ross, Thandi Sukhwinder, Brittain Clare, Kai Joe, Griffiths Frances, 'Acceptability of and Treatment Preferences For Recurrent Bacterial vaginosis—Topical Lactic Acid Gel or Oral Metronidazole Antibiotic: Qualitative Findings from the VITA trial'. *PLoS ONE*, Volume 14, Issue 11 (2019), p. e0224964. (Accessed 13 November 2020).

59. B. Andersch, D. Lindell, I. Dahlén and Å. Brandberg (1990). 'Bacterial vaginosis and the Effect of Intermittent Prophylactic Treatment with an Acid Lactate Gel'. *Gynecol. Obstet. Invest.*, Volume 31, Issue 2 (1990), pp. 114–119. doi: 10.1159/000293230 (Accessed 13 November 2020).

60. BioMedica Nutraceuticals, 'The Diverse Clinical Applications Of N-Acetyl-Cysteine: Technical Sheet'. Version 02/19 (2019).

61. S. Dinicola, S. De Grazia, G. Carlomagno and P. P. Pintucci, 'N-Acetylcysteine as Powerful Molecule to Destroy Bacterial Biofilms. A Systematic Review'. *European Review for Medical and Pharmacological Sciences*, Volume 18, Issue 19 (2014), pp. 2942–2948. PMID: 25339490 (Accessed 12 December 2020).

62. Michael Rotblatt and Irwin Zement, *Evidence-Based Herbal Medicine* (Philadelphia: Hanley & Belfus, Inc. Medical Publishers, 2002).

63. Ashwini Jadhav, Supriya Mortale, Shivkrupa Halbandge, Priyanka Jangid, Rajendra Patil, Wasudev Gade, Kiran Kharat and Sankunny Mohan Karuppayil, 'The Dietary Food Components Capric Acid and Caprylic Acid Inhibit Virulence Factors in *Candida albicans* Through Multitargeting'. *Journal of Medicinal Food*, Volume 20, Issue 11 (2017), pp. 1083–1090. doi: 10.1089/jmf.2017.3971 (Accessed 13 December 2020).

64. Joseph Mercola, 'Women Beware: Most Feminine Hygiene Products Contain Toxic Ingredients'. *HuffPost.* https://www.huffpost.com/entry/feminine-hygiene-products_b_3359581 (Accessed 11 January 2021).

65. M. Jaeger, A. Carvalho, C. Cunha, T. S. Plantinga, F. van de Veerdonk, M. Puccetti, C. Galosi, L. A. B Joosten, B. Dupont, B. J. Kullberg, J. D. Sobel, L. Romani and M. G. Netea, 'Association of a Variable Number Tandem Repeat in the NLRP3 Gene in Women with Susceptibility to RVVC'. *Eur. J. Clin. Microbiol. Infect. Dis.*, Volume 35 (2016), pp. 797–801. doi: 10.1007/s10096-016-2600-5 (Accessed 13 January 2021).

INDEX

abdominal massage, 114. *See also*
    therapeutics
  therapies, 189
ACV. *See* apple cider vinegar
adaptogens, 149
adolescence, 37–39
aerobic vaginitis (AV), 52, 185
    cautions, 53–54
    symptoms, 52–53
    test, 53
    treatment, 53
AFE spot, 83. *See also* orgasm
allergic conditions, 47
allergic contact dermatitis, 63–64
allopathic, 184
aloe vera, 120–121, 161. *See also*
    anti-fungal herbs; anti-
    inflammatory herbs
alterative, 184
amphoteric, 184
anaemia, megaloblastic, 146
anterior, 184
antibiotics, 75–76

anti-chaffing chamois, 171
anti-fungal herbs, 161. *See also*
    therapeutics
  aloe vera, 161
  caprylic acid, 163–164
  garlic, 161
  marigold, 161
  olive, 162–163
  oregano, 163
  p'au d'arco, 161–162
  thyme, 161
anti-inflammatory herbs, 119. *See also*
    therapeutics
  aloe vera, 120–121
  chamomile, 119–120
  green tea, 122
  marigold, 123–124
  sodium bicarbonate, 124
  witch hazel, 121–122
antimicrobial herbs, 155. *See also*
    therapeutics
  barberry, 155
  garlic, 157–158

lactic acid gel, 159–160
N-acetyl-cystine, 160–161
old man's beard, 156
probiotics as pessaries, 160
sodium bicarbonate, 161
thyme, 158
vitamin C, 159
antiviral herbs, 34
aphrodisiacs, 82, 140. *See also*
     intercourse; therapeutics
     ashwagandha, 142–143
     biotin, 145–146
     chamomile, 141
     cobalamin, 146–147
     damiana, 147–148
     folic acid, 146
     jasmine, 150–151
     mimosa, 149–150
     niacin, 144–145
     oats, 140–141
     pantothenic acid, 145
     pyridoxine, 145
     riboflavin, 144
     rose, 141–142
     saffron, 150–151
     Siberian ginseng, 148–149
     thiamin, 144
     vitamin B, 143–144
apple cider vinegar (ACV), 154–155.
     See also pH modulation
arousal, 79–81. *See also* intercourse
artificial oestrogens, 38
ascorbic acid. *See* vitamin C
ashwagandha, 142–143. *See also*
     aphrodisiacs; nervines
astringent, 184
atrophy, 184
AV. *See* aerobic vaginitis

bacterial imbalance, 42
bacterial infections, 35
bacterial vaginosis (BV), 43, 99, 185
     antibiotics, 45–46
     infection mode, 45
     symptoms, 44
     test, 44
     treatment, 44–45

balance, 15
     bacterial imbalance, 42
     of vagina, 14–15
barberry, 155. *See also* antimicrobial
     herbs
bayberry, 137–138. *See also* mucous
     membrane integrity
bearberry, 164–165. *See also* herbs for
     urinary problems
benzo[a]pyrene-diolepoxide (BPDE), 92
bicarbonate of soda. *See* sodium
     bicarbonate
bioavailable, 185
biofilms, 45
biologically fertile years, 39
     aerobic vaginitis, 52–54
     allergic contact dermatitis, 63–64
     antibiotics, 75–76
     bacterial imbalance, 42
     bacterial vaginosis, 43–46
     birth and post birth, 65–68
     clitoridynia, 58–61
     common conditions during, 43
     cystic glands, 58
     cytolytic vaginosis, 51–52
     fertile, 40
     fertility, 65–68
     irritant contact dermatitis, 62–63
     lichen planus, 56–57
     lichen sclerosus, 55–56
     miscarriage, 65–68
     mollicutes, 54–55
     neo-vagina and likely conditions, 78
     pain, 58–61
     pelvic congestion, 69–70
     pelvic congestion syndrome, 69
     pelvic inflammatory disease, 69
     periods, 39–41
     pH and testing, 41–42
     pregnancy, 65–68
     STIs, 70–75
     swabs, 42–43
     thrush, 46–51
     unclear symptoms, 76–78
     UTIs and urinary tract microbiome,
        68–69
     vaginal prolapse, 64–65

vaginismus, 61–62
vaginitis, 62
vestibulodynia, 58–61
vulvodynia, 58–61
biotin, 145–146. *See also* aphrodisiacs;
    nervines
birth
    caesarean birth, 66
    healing following birth, 67
    instrumental birth, 66
    mother-roasting or -warming, 67
    and post birth, 65–68
blended orgasm, 82. *See also* orgasm
blood glucose levels, 173–177. *See also*
    therapeutics
BPDE. *See* benzo[a]pyrene-diolepoxide
broadleaf plantain, 135–136. *See also*
    mucous membrane integrity
buchu, 166. *See also* herbs for urinary
    problems
BV. *See* bacterial vaginosis

caesarean birth, 66
Candida, 34–35
    albicans, xix
caprylic acid, 163–164. *See also*
    anti-fungal herbs
CBD infused, 191. *See also* menstrual
    wear selection
cervical. *See also* intercourse; orgasm
    health, 84–86
    orgasm, 83
    screenings, 84, 189
cervix, 84
    as source of pleasure, 86
chamomile, 119–120, 134, 141. *See also*
    anti-inflammatory herbs;
    aphrodisiacs; digestion and
    elimination herbs; nervines
childhood and pre-puberty, 30–31
    bacterial infections, 35
    Candida, 34–35
    consent, 36–37
    dermatological issues, 32
    good intimate health for female
        child, 36
    lichen sclerosis, 35

nappy rash, 31–32
pinworms, 33
poor hygiene, 33
presence of foreign bodies, 32
signs and diagnosis, 35–36
vaginal discharge from viral
    infections, 34
viruses, 33–34
vulvovaginal symptoms, 31
chlamydia, 72. *See also* sexually
    transmitted infections
chlorhexidine, 88. *See also* lubricants
chronic vulvovaginal candidiasis
    (CVVC), 185
cinnamon, 133–134. *See also* digestion
    and elimination herbs
clitoral orgasm, 82–83. *See also* orgasm
clitoridynia, 58–61
clitoris, xvii–xviii, 16–17. *See also* vulva
clothing, 169–170. *See also* therapeutics
cobalamin, 146–147. *See also*
    aphrodisiacs; nervines
colposcopy, 185
commensal microbes, 42
complex regional pain syndrome
    (CRPS), 59
compresses, 110–111. *See also*
    therapeutics
condoms, 90. *See also* intercourse
    resources, 187
congenital, 185
consent, 36–37. *See also* childhood and
    pre-puberty
contact dermatitis, irritant, 62–63
contraception, hormonal, 93
coping, 7
cornsilk, 165. *See also* herbs for urinary
    problems
cranberry, 167–168. *See also* herbs for
    urinary problems
cream, 113–114. *See also* therapeutics
Crone, 100
CRPS. *See* complex regional pain
    syndrome
CV. *See* cytolytic vaginosis
CVVC. *See* chronic vulvovaginal
    candidiasis

cystic glands, 58
cytolytic vaginosis (CV), 51, 185
　　cautions, 52
　　home pH test, 51–52
　　symptoms, 51
　　treatment, 52

damiana, 147–148. *See also*
　　　　aphrodisiacs; nervines
dandelion, 132–133. *See also* digestion
　　　　and elimination herbs
de-armouring, 83–86. *See also*
　　　　intercourse
decoctions, 108–109. *See also*
　　　　therapeutics
deinfibulation, 10
dental dams, 187
dermatitis
　　allergic contact, 63–64
　　irritant contact, 62–63
　　Lichen simplex chronicus, 63
　　treatment, 63–64
dermatological issues, 32. *See also*
　　　　childhood and pre-puberty
desquamative inflammatory vaginitis
　　　　(DIV), 53, 128
DHA. *See* docosahexaenoic acid
dietary impacts
　　on digestive health, 172
　　on immune health, 172–173
digestion and elimination herbs, 132.
　　　　See also therapeutics
　　chamomile, 134
　　cinnamon, 133–134
　　dandelion, 132–133
　　gut motility improvement, 134–135
　　senna, 135
digestive health, 172. *See also*
　　　　therapeutics
dilators, 188
dildos, 188
discs and cups, 190–191. *See also*
　　　　menstrual wear selection
DIV. *See* desquamative inflammatory
　　　　vaginitis

D-mannose, 168. *See also* herbs for
　　　　urinary problems
docosahexaenoic acid (DHA), 138
dosage forms, 107–108. *See also*
　　　　therapeutics
dynia, 58
dysbiosis, 23, 40, 185
dysgenesis, 27
dysplasia, 84–86. *See also* intercourse

Echinacea, 125–126. *See also* immunity
　　　　herbs
EFAs. *See* essential fatty acids
EFAs, 138–139. *See also* mucous
　　　　membrane integrity
EGCG. *See* epigallocatechin gallate
empirical, 185
endogenous, 185
　　oestrogen, 93
endorphins, 81
energetics, 114–115. *See also*
　　　　therapeutics
epigallocatechin gallate (EGCG), 122
episiotomy, 66
essential fatty acids (EFAs), 138
eubiotic/eubiosis, 185
excipient, 185
exogenous, 185
　　oestrogen, 38, 93
external female genitalia. *See* vulva
extrinsic factor, 146

Fanimesto, 2
fanny farts, 64
fatty acids, 139
female genital mutilation (FGM), 9
　　charities working to prevent, 191
　　complications, 10
　　deinfibulation, 10
　　types, 9
female neonate, 30
female reproductive system, 15
　　nerve bundles, 21–22
　　pelvic nerve, 21–22
　　pudendal nerve, 21–22

fennel, 151–152. *See also* hormonal
    herbs
fertility, 65–68
FGM. *See* female genital mutilation
folic acid, 146. *See also* aphrodisiacs;
    nervines
foreign bodies, 32. *See also* childhood
    and pre-puberty

galactagogue, 185
gammalinolenic acid (GLA), 138
garlic, 157–158, 161. *See also* anti-fungal
    herbs; antimicrobial herbs
gels, 113–114. *See also* therapeutics
genital area, 21
genitalia, external female. *See* vulva
genitourinary medicine (GUM), 70
GLA. *See* gammalinolenic acid
gladius, xvii
glans, 16. *See also* vulva
glycerine, 88. *See also* lubricants
gonorrhoea, 71. *See also* sexually
    transmitted infections
green tea, 122. *See also* anti-
    inflammatory herbs
G spot, 83. *See also* orgasm
guided mediation, 180–181. *See also*
    therapeutics
GUM. *See* genitourinary medicine
gut motility, 134–135. *See also* digestion
    and elimination herbs

Hart's Line, 18–19. *See also* vulva
hepatitis B, 73. *See also* sexually
    transmitted infections
herbs. *See also* therapeutics
    choosing, 107
    getting to know, 118
    retaking, 118
    stockists in UK, 189–190
    for urinary problems, 164–168
herbs for urinary problems, 164.
        See also therapeutics
    bearberry, 164–165
    buchu, 166

cornsilk, 165
cranberry, 167–168
D-mannose, 168
nettle, 166–167
UTIs, 168
herpes, 74. *See also* sexually transmitted
    infections
high vaginal swab, 42–43. *See also*
    biologically fertile years
hip baths, 110. *See also* therapeutics
histamine diet, low, 172. *See also*
    therapeutics
histamine intolerance, 172
HIV. *See* human immunodeficiency
    virus
homeostasis, 185
hormonal birth control, 93–94.
        See also intercourse
hormonal herbs, 151. *See also*
        therapeutics
    fennel, 151–152
    phyto-oestrogenic foods, 153
    red clover, 152–153
HPV. *See* human papilloma virus
human immunodeficiency virus
    (HIV), 72–73. *See also* sexually
    transmitted infections
human papilloma virus (HPV), 84–86.
        See also intercourse
hygiene, 33, 90–91, 169–170. *See also*
        childhood and pre-puberty;
        intercourse; therapeutics
hymen, 19–20. *See also* vulva

iatrogenic, 185
immune health, 92, 172–173. *See also*
        therapeutics
immunity herbs, 124. *See also*
        therapeutics
    Echinacea, 125–126
    maca, 131–132
    marigold, 124
    medicinal mushrooms, 124–125
    prebiotics, 129
    probiotic, 129–130

vitamin C, 126–127
vitamin D, 127–128
zinc, 130–131
infections, bacterial, 35
inflammation, 27
innervation, 185
instrumental birth, 66
intercourse, 79, 115
    aphrodisiacs, 82
    condoms, 90
    considerations, 86–93
    emotional component to vaginal
        health, 94
    hormonal birth control, 93–94
    hygiene, 90–91
    immune health, 92
    lubricants, 86–90
    menstrual protection, 92–93
    neo-vagina and penetrative sex,
        95–96
    obesity, 92
    orgasm, 81–84
    peeing after sex, 91
    sexual health status and testing, 86
    sexual response, 79–81
    smoking, 91–92
    as source of pleasure, 86
    toys, 90
    trauma, 94–95
    vaginal health and, 79
intrauterine system (IUS), 93
intrinsic factor, 146
irritant contact dermatitis, 62–63
IUS. *See* intrauterine system

jasmine, 150–151. *See also* aphrodisiacs;
    nervines

labia, 16. *See also* vulva
lactic acid gel, 159–160. *See also*
    antimicrobial herbs
Lactobacillus, 93
    overgrowth syndrome. *See* cytolytic
        vaginosis
    species, 23–24
leucorrhea, 38, 185. *See also* vaginal
    discharge

libido, 79–81. *See also* intercourse
lichen planus (LP), 56–57
lichen sclerosus (LS), 35, 55–56
LP. *See* lichen planus
LS. *See* lichen sclerosus
lubricants, 86. *See also* intercourse
    ingredients in, 87–89
    resources, 188
    selection, 89–90
    types, 90
lymph nodes, 69

maca, 131–132. *See also* immunity herbs
Mage stage, 100
Maiden, 100
marc, 185
marigold, 123–124, 161. *See also*
        anti-fungal herbs; anti-
        inflammatory herbs;
        immunity herbs
marshmallow root, 137. *See also*
        mucous membrane integrity
Materia Medica, 114, 116. *See also*
        therapeutics
    choosing remedies, 116–117
mediation, 185
medical herbalists, 188
medicinal mushrooms, 124–125.
        See also immunity herbs
megaloblastic anaemia, 146
menarche, 37
menopause
    peri-menopause into, 96
    into post-menopausal, 97–101
menopause into post-menopausal
        changes, 97
    freedom and power, 100–101
    in microbiome, 99–100
    in vagina, 98–99
    vaginismus, 98
menstrual blood, 24
menstrual protection, 92–93. *See also*
        intercourse
menstrual wear selection, 190. *See also*
        periodwear
    CBD infused, 191
    discs and cups, 190–191

period pants, 190
reusable cloth pads, 191
sustainable organic disposables,
    190
menstruum, 185
Metronidazole, 45
micro, 25
microbiome testing kit, 78
mimosa, 149–150. *See also* aphrodisiacs;
    nervines
mineral oils and derivatives, 88.
    See also lubricants
miscarriage, 65–68
mollicutes, 54–55
molluscum contagiosum, 75. *See
    also* sexually transmitted
    infections
mons, 16. *See also* vulva
Mother, 100
mother-roasting or -warming, 67
mucous membrane integrity, 135.
    See also therapeutics
    bayberry, 137–138
    broadleaf plantain, 135–136
    EFAs, 138–139
    marshmallow root, 137
    sea buckthorn oil, 140
myco, 26

NAC. *See* n-acetyl-cystine
N-acetyl-cystine (NAC), 160–161. *See
    also* antimicrobial herbs
nappy rash, 31–32. *See also* childhood
    and pre-puberty
natal vaginas, 27–28
naturopaths, 188
neo-vaginas, 9, 27–28. *See also* vagina
    adequate sexual functionality, 95
    and likely conditions, 78
    and penetrative sex, 95–96
nervines, 140. *See also* therapeutics
    ashwagandha, 142–143
    biotin, 145–146
    chamomile, 141
    cobalamin, 146–147
    damiana, 147–148
    folic acid, 146

jasmine, 150–151
mimosa, 149–150
niacin, 144–145
oats, 140–141
pantothenic acid, 145
pyridoxine, 145
riboflavin, 144
rose, 141–142
saffron, 150–151
Siberian ginseng, 148–149
thiamin, 144
vitamin B, 143–144
nettle, 166–167. *See also* herbs for
    urinary problems
niacin, 144–145. *See also* aphrodisiacs;
    nervines
nociception, 185
nonoxynol 9, 88. *See also* lubricants
nutritional therapists, 189

oats, 140–141. *See also* aphrodisiacs;
    nervines
obesity, 92. *See also* intercourse
octanoic acid. *See* caprylic acid
octoxynol 9, 88. *See also* lubricants
oestrogen, 26
    artificial, 38
    circulating, 30
    endogenous, 93
    exogenous, 38
    exogenous, 93
    level drop, 98
    types of, 96
ointments, 113–114. *See also*
    therapeutics
old man's beard, 156. *See also*
    antimicrobial herbs
olive, 162–163. *See also* anti-fungal
    herbs
omega 3 oils, 139
omega 7, 140
oophorectomy, 185
oregano, 163. *See also* anti-fungal
    herbs
organic foods, 173
orgasm, 81–84. *See also* intercourse
    AFE spot, 83

blended, 82
cervical, 83
clitoral, 82–83
G spot, 83
neurotransmitters released at, 81
toys, 84–85
Os, 185
oxytocin, 81

pain windup, 59
pantothenic acid, 145. *See also*
    aphrodisiacs; nervines
pap test, 84–85
parabens, 88. *See also* lubricants
p'au d'arco, 161–162. *See also*
    anti-fungal herbs
PCS. *See* pelvic congestion syndrome
peeing after sex, 91. *See also* intercourse
pelvic. *See also* therapeutics
    congestion, 69–70
    health physio, 179
    health physiotherapists, 189
    nerve, 21–22
    organs, 64
pelvic congestion syndrome (PCS), 69
pelvic inflammatory disease (PID), 69
penetrative sex, 95–96
peri-menopause, 96
    into menopause, 96–97
perineum, 18. *See also* vulva
period pants, 190. *See also* menstrual
    wear selection
periods, 39–41. *See also* biologically
    fertile years
periodwear, 170–171. *See also*
    therapeutics
peristalsis, 186
pessaries, 112. *See also* therapeutics
    marigold, 123
    probiotics as, 154, 160
    vitamin C, 159
pH. *See also* biologically fertile years
    modulation, 153–155
    and testing, 41–42
    test strips, 153–154
phase, 186

pH modulation, 153. *See also*
    therapeutics
    apple cider vinegar, 154–155
    probiotics as pessaries, 154
phthalates, 88. *See also* lubricants
phytochemicals, 108
phytoestrogens, 153
phyto-oestrogenic foods, 153. *See also*
    hormonal herbs
PID. *See* pelvic inflammatory disease
pinworms, 33. *See also* childhood and
    pre-puberty
pleasure, 84–86. *See also* intercourse
    tools, 188
polyquaternium 15, 88. *See also* lubricants
posterior, 186
post-menopausal
    chnge, 97–101
    vagina, 98
potentiate, 186
prebiotics, 129. *See also* immunity herbs
pre-cancerous cell change, 85
pregnancy, 65–68
    episiotomy, 66
pre-menarch, 37–39
probiotic, 129–130. *See also*
    antimicrobial herbs; immunity
    herbs; pH modulation
    as pessaries, 154, 160
professional practitioner bodies, 188
    abdominal massage therapies, 189
    medical herbalists, 188
    naturopaths, 188
    nutritional therapists, 189
    pelvic health physiotherapists, 189
    psychological therapies, 189
    somatic and sexual therapists, 189
progesterone, 26
prolactin, 81
prolapse, vaginal, 64–65
propylene glycol, 89. *See also* lubricants
psychological therapies, 189
pubic. *See also* sexually transmitted
    infections; therapeutics
    hair, 170
    lice, 73

pudendal nerve, 21–22
pyridoxine, 145. *See also* aphrodisiacs;
    nervines

recurrent vulvovaginal candidiasis
    (RVVC), 186
red clover, 152–153. *See also* hormonal
    herbs
resources, 187
    abdominal massage therapies, 189
    CBD infused, 191
    charities to prevent FGM, 191
    condoms, 187
    dental dams, 187
    discs and cups, 190–191
    glass, ceramic and body-safe crystal
        dildos, 188
    herb stockists in the UK, 189–190
    intimate lubricants, 188
    medical herbalists, 188
    menstrual wear selection, 190–191
    naturopaths, 188
    nutritional therapists, 189
    pelvic health physiotherapists,
        189
    for people with cervical screenings,
        189
    period pants, 190
    pleasure tools, 188
    professional practitioner bodies,
        188–189
    psychological therapies, 189
    reusable cloth pads, 191
    sexual health screening, 187
    somatic and sexual therapists, 189
    supplements and products for self-
        guided purchase, 190
    sustainable organic disposables,
        190
    therapists, 192
    vibrating dilators for vaginismus,
        188
reusable cloth pads, 191. *See also*
    menstrual wear selection
riboflavin, 144. *See also* aphrodisiacs;
    nervines

rose, 141–142. *See also* aphrodisiacs;
    nervines
rowing and cycling, 171. *See also*
    therapeutics
RVVC. *See* recurrent vulvovaginal
    candidiasis

saffron, 150–151. *See also* aphrodisiacs;
    nervines
sea buckthorn oil, 140. *See also* mucous
    membrane integrity
senna, 135. *See also* digestion and
    elimination herbs
serotonin, 81
sex, 115–116. *See also* therapeutics
    penetrative, 95–96
sexual functionality, adequate, 95
sexual health. *See also* intercourse
    screening, 187
    status and testing, 86
sexually transmitted infections (STIs),
    49, 70–75
    chlamydia, 72
    common, 71–75
    gonorrhoea, 71
    hepatitis B, 73
    herpes, 74
    HIV, 72–73
    molluscum contagiosum, 75
    pubic lice, 73
    self-care, 70
    syphilis, 71–72
    trichomoniasis, 74
sexual response, 79–81. *See also*
    intercourse
shammy' creams, 171
Siberian ginseng, 148–149. *See also*
    aphrodisiacs; nervines
Simples, 110, 186
sitz bath and washes, 110. *See also*
    therapeutics
smears, 84–86. *See also* intercourse
smoking, 91–92. *See also* intercourse
sodium bicarbonate, 89, 124, 161. *See*
    also anti-inflammatory herbs;
    antimicrobial herbs

sodium hydroxide, 89. *See also* lubricants
somatic and sexual therapists, 189
somatise, 186
squirting, 83. *See also* orgasm
steams, 111. *See also* therapeutics
steroid hormones, 139
STIs. *See* sexually transmitted infections
sugar, 175
    substitutes, 176
supplements and products for self-guided purchase, 190
supportive supplements, 176
suppositories, 112. *See also* therapeutics
sustainable organic disposables, 190. *See also* menstrual wear selection
symptoms, unclear, 76–78
synthetic dyes, 89. *See also* lubricants
synthetic fragrances, 89. *See also* lubricants
syphilis, 71–72. *See also* sexually transmitted infections
systemic, 186

tea, 108–109. *See also* therapeutics
testosterone, 26
therapeutics, 105, 181–182
    abdominal massage, 114
    aggravated symptoms, 118
    anti-fungal herbs, 161–164
    anti-inflammatory herbs, 119–124
    antimicrobial herbs, 155–161
    blood glucose levels, 173–177
    choosing herbs, 107
    compresses, 110–111
    creative expression, 178–179
    dietary impacts health, 172–173
    digestion and elimination herbs, 132–135
    dosage forms, 107–108
    energetics, 114–115
    getting to know herbs, 118
    guided mediation to help connection with vagina, 180–181
    herbs for urinary problems, 164–168
    hierarchy of, 117–118
    hormonal herbs, 151–153
    hygiene, clothing and toilet paper, 169–170
    immunity herbs, 124–132
    journaling prompts, 177–178
    lifestyle considerations, 169
    limitations, 106–107
    low histamine diet, 172
    Materia Medica, 116–117
    minimising disruption to intimate ecology, 171
    mucous membrane integrity, 135–140
    nervines and aphrodisiacs, 140–151
    pelvic health physio, 179
    periodwear, 170–171
    pessaries, 112
    pH modulation, 153–155
    pubic hair, 170
    rowing and cycling, 171
    sex, 115–116
    singing, 178
    sitz bath and washes, 110
    steams, 111
    taking herbs, 118
    tea and decoctions, 108–109
    tincture, 109
    topical preparations, 113–114
    vaginal dilators, 173
    working topically with vagina, 112–113
therapists, 192
thiamin, 144. *See also* aphrodisiacs; nervines
three ages of womanhood, 100
thrush, 40, 42, 46. *See also* vulvovaginal candidiasis
    cautions, 49
    chronic, 47
    infection mode, 47–48
    recurrent thrush, 47
    symptoms, 46
    test, 46
    treatment, 48–50

thyme, 158, 161. *See also* anti-fungal herbs; antimicrobial herbs
thymoleptic, 186
tincture, 109. *See also* therapeutics
tisanes. *See* tea
toilet paper, 169–170. *See also* therapeutics
topical. *See also* therapeutics
    anti-inflamm atory herbs, 48
    preparations, 113–114
toxic shock syndrome (TSS), 69
toys, 90. *See also* intercourse
    resources, 188
traditional Western herbal medicine, 107. *See also* therapeutics
trauma, 94–95
trichomoniasis, 74. *See also* sexually transmitted infections
triclosan, 89. *See also* lubricants
triglycerides, 139
TSS. *See* toxic shock syndrome

urethral opening, 18. *See also* vulva
urethral sponge, 18
urinary tract infections (UTIs), 68–69, 168. *See also* herbs for urinary problems
urinary tract microbiome, 68–69
UTIs. *See* urinary tract infections

vagina, 2, 8, 19. *See also* neo-vagina; therapeutics; thrush; vulva
    acupuncture point, 3
    atrophy, 151
    balance of, 14–15
    candidiasis. *See* thrush
    cervix, 8
    changes in microbiome, 99–100
    diet for health of, 6
    dilators, 173
    etymology of, xvii
    external female genitalia, 14
    female genital mutilation, 9–11
    health care provider about vaginal health, 6–7
    hormones, 26–27
    maintenance, 6

moisturisers, 98
mycobiome, 25–26
natal, 27–28
neo-vaginas, 9, 27–28
prolapse, 64–65
smell, 21
social norms, 8–9
thrush infections, xix
vaginal microbiome, 23–25
virobiome, 26
vulva, 8
working topically with, 112–113
vaginal discharge, 7, 20, 38. *See also* vulva
    from viral infections, 34
vaginal health, 182
    diet for, 6
    emotional component to, 94
    health care provider about, 6–7
    hormonal contraception, 93
    intercourse, 79
    symptoms, 7
    talking to partners about, 101–104
vaginal microbiome, 23–24, 38, 78
    changes in, 99–100
    cyclical changes to, 24–25
    Lactobacillus species, 23–24
    tests, 25
vaginal prolapse, 64–65
vaginismus, 61–62
    resources, 188
vaginitis, 62
    aerobic, 52–54
vaginocele, 64
vaginosis, cytolytic, 51–52
vestibular bulbs, 21
vestibule, 16–18. *See also* vulva
vestibulodynia, 58–61
viruses, 33–34
vitamin B, 143–144. *See also* aphrodisiacs; nervines
vitamin C (ascorbic acid), 126–127, 159. *See also* immunity herbs
vitamin D, 127–128. *See also* immunity herbs
vulva, 14, 16. *See also* female genital mutilation

clitoris, 16–17
glans, 16
Hart's Line, 18–19
hymen, 19–20
innervation, 21–22
labia, 16
mons, 16
mucosa and discharge, 20
pelvic nerve, 21–22
perineum, 18
pudendal nerve, 21–22
smell, 21
urethral opening, 18
urethral sponge, 18
vagina, 19
vestibule, 17–18
vestibule area, 16
vulval skin, 18

vulvodynia, 58–61
    cautions, 60
    pain windup, 59
    symptoms, 59
    treatments, 60
vulvovaginal candidiasis (VVC), 38, 46,
        186. *See* vaginal health
VVC. *See* vulvovaginal candidiasis

wet mount. *See* high vaginal swab
whiff test, 44
Wickham's Stria, 56
witch hazel, 121–122. *See also* anti-
        inflammatory herbs
womanhood, three ages of, 100

zinc, 130–131. *See also* immunity herbs

CPSIA information can be obtained
at www.ICGtesting.com
Printed in the USA
JSHW040528080922
30131JS00001B/1

9 781913 504885